Clinics in Human Lactation

The Nipple and Areola in Breastfeeding and Lactation

Anatomy, Physiology, Problems, and Solutions

By Marsha Walker, RN, IBCLC

The Nipple and Areola in Breastfeeding and Lactation

Anatomy, Physiology, Problems, and Solutions

Marsha Walker, RN, IBCLC

Praeclarus Press, LLC
2504 Sweetgum Lane
Amarillo, Texas 79124 USA
806-367-9950
www.PraeclarusPress.com

DISCLAIMER
The information contained in this publication is advisory only and is not intended to replace sound clinical judgment or individualized patient care. The author disclaims all warranties, whether expressed or implied, including any warranty as the quality, accuracy, safety, or suitability of this information for any particular purpose.

ISBN: 9781939807724

Table of Contents

Section 1

Anatomy and Physiology

INTRODUCTION

The nipple and areola represent the point of interaction between the infant and the breast, forming a conduit through which breastmilk passes on its path to the infant. These structures act as a "handle" or the contact point used by the infant to grasp the breast and engage in sucking motions that result in the transfer of milk from the breast to the infant's mouth. Their multifaceted roles in mother/infant interactions include protective, mechanical, communicative, and nurturing. They have been evolutionarily shaped to optimize mother/infant co-adaptation.

Most animals have areas on their skin where the epidermis is specialized to serve as an interface with the environment. These areas of specialized epidermis are characterized by reduced numbers of hairs (or feathers or scales), specific patterns of cell differentiation, and adaptation to changing states within the animal. They express distinctive keratins that provide an increased ability to withstand mechanical strain (Eastwood et al., 2007). Keratins are structural proteins of epidermal cells that act as a resilient scaffold, permitting epithelial cells to function under mechanical stresses. The nipple has a type of specialized epidermis that is adapted to function under the mechanical strain of breastfeeding or nursing.

ANATOMY

Fetal Development

Breast development starts during the fourth week of gestation with the formation of a symmetrical ectodermal thickening along the ventral lateral sides of the embryo. Growth of a milk streak, milk lines, or ventral epidermal ridges is seen by the sixth week of gestation. During the second and third embryonic months, the glandular elements of the breasts are formed near the fourth and fifth ribs, with regression of the rest of the thickened ectodermal streaks. Alterations in breast and nipple development can occur if the epidermal ridges do not completely recede. Some foci may remain that can result in the development of polythelia - accessory or supernumerary nipples. The prevalence of accessory nipples is approximately 0.22–6% of the population, with differing populations showing distinct variations based on ethnicity, geographic location, and method used to determine accessory nipples (**Table 1-1**).

Table 1-1. Distribution of Accessory or Supernumerary Nipples Among Selected Populations

Population	Prevalence	Source
White American neonates	0.6%	Kenney, Flippo, & Black, 1987
White Europeans	0.22%	Mathes et al., 2006
African Americans	1.6%	Rahbar, 1982
Israeli children	2.5%	Mimouni, Merlob, & Reisner, 1983
Arab children	4.7%	Jaber & Merlob, 1988
Japanese women	5%	Johnson, Felson, & Jolles, 1986

The most common location for accessory nipples is on the milk line just below the breast, but supernumerary nipples can form anywhere along the milk lines. These extra nipples are often mistaken for a mole. Sometimes they may be differentiated enough to become active during lactation and may swell or secrete milk. Although they usually occur as a solitary anomaly, women can have more than one. Supernumerary nipples are benign, but are affected by the same hormonal changes and disease processes that affect normal breast tissue. If glandular tissue accompanies the accessory nipple, they can enlarge, swell, and become tender premenstrually, as well as produce milk during lactation. They have also been associated with a number of medical conditions, including an identified relationship with kidney and urinary tract malformations (Ferrara et al., 2009).

The frequency of urinary tract and renal defects in the general population is 1-2% (Cellini & Offidani, 1992). In patients with supernumerary nipples who have been evaluated with ultrasound, the frequency of kidney and urinary tract anomalies jumps to 14.5% (Varsano et al, 1984). If the supernumerary nipple is familial (runs in families), the frequency of kidney and urinary tract defects rises to approximately 30% (Casey, Chasan, & Chick, 1996). There are differing gradations or variations of supernumerary nipples. Kajava (1915) proposed a supernumerary nipple classification system that is still in use today (**Table 1-2**) (Brown & Schwartz, 2003).

Table 1-2. Kajava's Supernumerary Nipple Classification System

Classification	Description
1	Complete supernumerary nipple: contains a nipple, areola, and glandular tissue; called polymastia
2	Supernumerary nipple with glandular tissue, but without an areola
3	An areola and glandular tissue without a nipple
4	Glandular tissue only
5	Supernumerary nipple, areola, and pseudomamma (fat tissue that has replaced the glandular tissue)
6	Supernumerary nipple only; called polythelia; this is the most common type
7	Areola only (called polythelia areolaris)
8	Patch of hair only (called polythelia pilosa)

Adapted from (Kajava, 1915).

Treatment of a supernumerary nipple is usually unnecessary; however, it can be surgically removed if it causes the mother distress or discomfort from tenderness or lactation.

Appearance of the Nipple and Areola

The shape, size, and color of nipples and areolae vary greatly from mother to mother. Nipples may be large or inconspicuous, cylindrical or bifurcated, while the areola can be neatly circumscribed or diffusely pigmented, and small or large. This great variation is considered a genetic expression (Montagna & MacPherson, 1974). There can also be an appreciable difference between the two nipple-areola complexes in the same mother. Wide variability exists relative to the normal dimensions of the nipple/areola complex. In general, the reference B-C cup breast has an areola diameter of 4.2 to 5 cm, with the nipple diameter and height equal to one-third to one-fourth of the areola diameter. While the mean diameter of the areola is 4 cm, its size can range from 2.0–7.0 cm (Mathes, Seyfer, & Miranda, 2006). The average projection and size of human female nipples is slightly more than three-eighths of an inch (10mm). Pregnancy and nursing tend to increase nipple size, sometimes permanently. The central position of the nipple in the areola is variable, ranging from one-fourth to one-half of the radius off-center.

Nipple projection results from the primary location of the mammary ducts in the central portion of the nipple complex. This arrangement produces a semi-rigid structure with a significantly more fibrotic element than the soft, pliable surrounding areola. The contractile properties of the areola also contribute to the gradual change in nipple projection obtained with direct or neural stimuli. The color of both structures may range from light pink or light brown in fair skinned women to dark brown or black in women with dark hair or mothers of color. The pigment melanin, which is responsible for skin and hair color in mammals, is produced in specialized cells called melanocytes, and then distributed to other cells. The pigments of the nipple and areola are brown eumelanin (a brown pigment) and to a greater extent pheomelanin (a red pigment). The amount of melanin in areolar and nipple skin is more than twice that found in the surrounding breast skin, which gives the nipple/areolar complex its darker color (Dean et al., 2005).

Melanin has many functions that include protection from ultraviolet rays and helping the skin resist abrasion. One of the early signs of pregnancy is darkening of the nipples and areolae. During pregnancy there is an increase in melanin formation, with a greater number of pregnancies causing progressive darkening of the nipple/areola, showing a cumulative retention of pigmentation. Increased melanocyte stimulating activity has been found in the blood and urine of pregnant women (Robins, 1991). Differences in nipple/areola color exist among black, white, oriental, and Native American mothers, with white mothers tending to have the lightest areolae, black mothers tending to have the darkest, and Asian and Native American mothers somewhere in between (Pawson & Petrakis, 1975). There is no apparent relationship between nipple pigmentation and nipple soreness or damage during breastfeeding. Fair-skinned mothers do not experience more nipple soreness or cracking than do darker-skinned mothers, even though their nipples and areolae may be much lighter (Gans, 1958; Brown & Hurlock, 1975; Hewat & Ellis, 1987; Ziemer, Paone, Schupay, & Cole, 1990).

The tip of the nipple is characterized by a dense cluster of papillar-like elevations or protuberances with unique patterns of crevices and nipple pore openings. The sides of the nipple contain intersecting grooves which permit the nipple to flatten when not erect. There are no hairs on the nipple or areola, but the outer border of the areola is ringed by hairs.

The Glands of Montgomery

The nipple and areola are densely supplied with various types of skin glands. The areolar tubercles that surround the nipple represent the ducts of Montgomery and sebaceous glands (oil-secreting glands) and are usually found together throughout the areola. The tubercles vary in size, number, and pattern of distribution. There are between 1-15 Montgomery gland tubercles on the areola of about 1-2 mm in size. They may enlarge during pregnancy and become quite prominent. The ducts of the sebaceous glands often empty near or into the ducts of the Montgomery glands. The ducts and sinuses of the Montgomery apparatus are richly vascularized and innervated and often become functional during lactation. They represent true mammary glands surrounded by nerve fibers, capillaries, and delicate elastic fibers (Montagna & Yun, 1972). Some sweat glands also open onto the areola.

Because the glands of Montgomery have a secretory apparatus and capacity, they have the potential to become obstructed. The ductal system of the areola can also become inflamed or infected (Al-Qattan & Robertson, 1990; Blech, Friebe, & Krause, 2004). A mother can experience a painful inflamed or infected Montgomery gland, which appears as a reddened raised bump or fluid-filled blister farther back on the areola. Although the condition is usually self-limiting, it can occasionally require interventions, such as the application of warm compresses, the use of antibiotics (topical or systemic), and gentle squeezing to remove infected material. Mothers should be aware of equipment or irritants that could precipitate or aggravate Montgomery glands to the point of actual obstruction or damage. Use of pump flanges, breast shells, or nipple shields that can abrade these glands or the application of topical preparations that can block the openings of the Montgomery glands should be investigated when mothers present with painful conditions on the areola rather than the nipple.

The Role of Scent in Early Breastfeeding

Schaal et al. (2006) described the areolar glandular system as having potential communicative, mechanical, and protective functions that include the following:

Olfactory Properties

Secretions from apocrine and eccrine sweat glands on the areola, sebaceous glands, and Montgomery glands mix with milk released from the nipple to form an odor-emitting mélange of substances that function as a chemoattractant to the infant. Neonates are responsive to odors naturally released from lactating breasts (Macfarlane, 1975; Makin & Porter, 1989; Russell, 1976; Schaal, 1986; Varendi et al., 1994). Porter & Winberg (1999) describe how a mother's breast odors elicit preferential head turning by newborns within minutes of birth that function as a guide toward the nipple. This is similar to nipple-search pheromones released by nonhuman mammals. They state that the chemical profile of areolar and nipple secretions may overlap with amniotic fluid, presenting the infant with a familiar odor which helps to further orient the infant to the breast. Infants learn to recognize their mother by her unique scent (Schaal et al., 2009) alone, which may be an important contributor in the development of the mother/infant bond.

Doucet et al. (2007) attempted to sort out the sources of active volatile compounds released by the lactating breast. Three-to-four-day old infants were presented the breast in a number of conditions: a scentless condition (entirely covered with a transparent film), nipple only exposed, areola only exposed, and milk exposed. The infants were more orally active when facing any of the odorous conditions of the breast as compared to the scentless condition. They cried earlier and longer and opened their eyes less when exposed to the scentless breast, showing that the release of volatile compounds in the areolar and milk secretions released mouthing, stimulated eye opening, and delayed and reduced crying. Breastmilk odor has a calming effect on infants as evidenced by their reduced crying and lower cortisol levels when exposed to their own mother's milk odor compared to another mother's milk, formula, or no exposure prior to a heel stick procedure (Nishitani et al., 2009).

Olfactory Enhancing Properties

The areola has a higher surface temperature compared to the nipple and breast due to the presence of Haller's subareolar vascular plexus (Mitz & Lalardie, 1977). This higher temperature enhances the evaporation of the odorants, improving their effectiveness as a chemical attractant. This feature of the areola is triggered by the crying of the infant (Vuorenkoski et al., 1969), resulting in maximum odor release when the infant goes to breast.

Protective Properties of the Lipid Fraction of Glandular Secretions

Sebum, a fatty secretion from sebaceous glands and Montgomery's tubercles, may act as an odor fixative that stabilizes the olfactory mixture of substances formed on the surface of the areola. It may also function as a lubricant to reduce mechanical stress on the nipple/areola and to protect the epidermis from factors in the infant's saliva that may break down tissue (Perkins & Miller, 1926). The areolar glands increase their activity during pregnancy and lactation, which may help protect the nipple/areolar epidermis and ductal openings from pathogens.

Properties to Enhance Sucking Effectiveness

The glandular secretions of the areola and nipple may combine with the infant's own saliva to improve the seal on the breast for effective vacuum generation (Epstein, Blass, Batshaw, & Parks, 1970). Increased numbers of Montgomery glands were shown to be associated with higher infant weight gain during the first three days after birth, less of a weight loss during the first three days, increased latching speed and sucking intensity, and decreased time to onset of lactation in first time mothers (Schaal et al., 2006). Thus, a higher population of Montgomery glands appeared to directly affect the newborn's behavior at the breast. With infants latching more easily and sucking more intensely, efficient colostrum intake would be expected and concomitant reduction in weight loss would be seen. More efficient nipple stimulation would contribute to timely lactogenesis II and a positive breastfeeding experience for the mother, reinforcing her confidence in herself.

Doucet, Soussignan, Sagot, and Schaal (2009) presented newborn infants with odor substrates collected directly from Montgomery glands and compared infant responses to other substrates including human milk, vanilla, infant formula, and cow's milk. Odor substrates from Montgomery glands presented under the newborns' noses elicited significantly increased amounts of head turning, lip pursing, tongue protrusion, and greater reactivity than any of the other substrates. The Montgomery-gland odor elicited immediate motor and respiratory responses of high amplitude during the time it was presented compared with all of the other odors, which showed a lower magnitude of responses that were also slower to appear. The volatile compounds from the Montgomery glands reliably activated behavioral and autonomic responses in newborns that favored enhanced breastfeeding.

The Importance of Keeping Mothers and Babies Together

These studies reinforce the importance of keeping mothers and infants together skin-to-skin so that these odor stimuli enhance the intake of colostrum and strengthen the maternal/infant bond. When an infant is held skin-to-skin between the breasts and in close proximity to the nipple/areolar complex, important feeding cues are presented to the infant in the early days, which would otherwise be missed if the infant is placed in a bassinet. Breast olfactory signals activate oral activity on the nipple and start a procession of behavioral processes that include neural, neuroendocrine, and endocrine functions in both the infant and the mother.

It is important that areolar secretions not be washed or wiped off or masked by preparations applied to the nipple/areola in the first few days following birth. Routine application of creams or ointments to the nipples in the early days should be avoided. Such practices may eliminate an important olfactory stimulus necessary to facilitate an optimal start to breastfeeding.

Nerves and Muscles in the Areola and Nipple

The nipple and areola are active participants in the breastfeeding process. The smooth muscle in the nipple and areola when contracted causes the areola to wrinkle and the nipple to stiffen and become erect. Montagna (1970) notes that most of the muscles converge towards the nipple and appear in a radial and circular arrangement. The longitudinal muscle bundles are most prominent in the center of the nipple where they course with the lactiferous ducts. These muscle bundles allow the nipple to become erect with stimulation. The connective tissue in the nipple has extensive elastic properties. Elastic fibers are most abundant under the epidermis at the tip of the nipple and surrounding the lactiferous ducts. Elastic fibers surround smooth muscle fibers, forming a fibrous support system for them and anchoring them to the surrounding tissue.

Nerves from branches of the second through fifth intercostal nerves innervate the nipple and areola. The extent of the contribution of each nerve is variable and can differ between breasts on the same woman (Sarhadi, Shaw, Lee, & Soutar, 1996). Nerves within the nipple are concentrated in the middle and move forward to the tip along the milk ducts. Few nerves are seen in the sides of the nipple or on the underside of the areola. Small nerve-end organs are seen at the nipple tip around the milk ducts and in the dermis underneath the grooves and crevices of the dermis. The milk ducts in the nipple are encircled throughout their length by loosely wrapped small and large nerve fibers.

The nipple is richly innervated with nerve fibers containing neuropeptide Y and tyrosine hydroxylase, which may be related to the role that the sympathetic nervous system plays in nipple erection (Eriksson, Lindh, Uvnas-Moberg, & Hokfelt, 1996). The epidermis of the nipple contains abundant innervation of nerve fibers containing vasoactive intestinal polypeptide, calcitonin gene-related peptide, and substance P, which are peptides known to influence muscle tone and may also have a role in the control of nipple erection (Uvnas-Moberg & Eriksson, 1996). The tip of the nipple contains many capillaries that become progressively shallower and sparser on the sides of the nipple, the areola, and the periareolar surface. Branches of the external and internal mammary arteries provide most of the blood supply to the nipple/areolar complex.

Ductal Network

The classic work on breast anatomy was conducted by Sir Astley Cooper in 1840 (Cooper, 1840). His cadaver dissections of lactating breasts revealed 7 to 12 patent ducts (ducts that actually drained lobes of the breast) in the nipple, although he could cannulate (insert a catheter) in as many as 22 ducts (**Figure 1-1**).

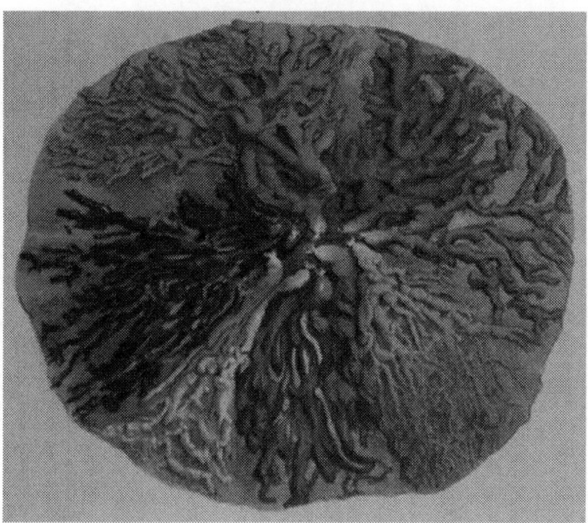

Figure 1-1. Wax-Injected Ductal System in Cadaver Dissection
From (Cooper, 1840).

Older textbooks describe 15–25 ductal openings on the tip of the nipple; however, direct observation, three-dimensional computer modeling, ultrasound, ductography, and actual dissections of the nipple have helped clarify and correct descriptions of its internal structure.

The following studies over the years have greatly improved our understanding of the internal structure of the nipple. Each study contributed a little more to the understanding of the complexity of the ductal structure of the nipple and breast. Differing study modalities did not always provide consistent results, but the general description of the size, number, and arrangement of nipple ducts have became clear in the later studies.

Duct Distribution

Duct distribution was studied in necropsy breasts through 2 mm sections in a study by Moffat and Going (1996). These researchers showed that each duct system drained a differing amount of breast tissue. These same researchers (Going & Moffat, 2004) described an autopsied breast through the use of 2-mm sections that showed seven ducts extended to the surface of the nipple, while 27 other ducts were present in the nipple, but terminated or disappeared into a skin appendage before they reached the nipple tip. Thus, the number of ducts in the nipple was much greater than the number of openings on the nipple tip, typically six to eight. The authors thought that this may occur due to bifurcation or branching of milk ducts close to the skin of the nipple or may represent two different duct populations, e.g., true milk ducts and ducts derived from skin appendages. One main collecting duct and its branches drained up to 23% of the total breast volume; the largest three systems drained 50%, and the largest six systems drained 75% of the breast. They liken the human breast to not one gland but many, with the lobes or ductal systems as separate domains.

Nipple Pores or Openings

Using computer-assisted reconstruction of 2 mm sections of breast tissue, Ohtake et al. (2001) showed that different lobular systems could occasionally be connected to each other (anastomoses between ducts of different lobes) and demonstrated several connections within the same lobular system. Love and Barsky (2004) used six different approaches to determine the number, distribution, and anatomic properties of the breast ductal system to resolve some of the inconsistencies in earlier research. Numerous indentations were observed on the tip of the nipple, with slightly under 10% associated with either sebaceous glands or sweat or apocrine ducts. Between five and nine actual ductal orifices or true lactiferous duct openings (nipple pores) were observed.

The pattern of orifices was described as a central orifice in the center of the nipple, a second orifice oriented in the upper, outer quadrant of the nipple, with a group of central orifices just above or below the central and other peripheral openings in the upper lateral, upper medial, and lower lateral quadrants the most common. There appeared to be two sets of ducts in the nipple, a central collection of ducts and a more peripheral group. The central ducts travel back from the nipple toward the chest wall, while the peripheral ducts drape over the central ducts in a radial fashion. Separate ductal systems may lie in the same breast quadrant and overlap each other, but these researchers saw no connections between systems.

Absence of Lactiferous Sinuses

Ramsay, Kent, Hartmann, and Hartmann (2005) used ultrasound to measure and describe the characteristics of the main portion of the ductal system, such as duct diameter, branching of the ducts, and their location in the breast. Ultrasound is able to detect ducts above 0.5 mm in diameter. The average number of main ducts greater than 0.5 mm in diameter at the base of the nipple was nine, with a range of 4 to 18. Duct diameters ranged from 1.0 to 4.4 mm at the base of the nipple, with an increase in diameter where ducts branched.

While there appeared to be no sacs, or "lactiferous sinuses," these widened areas under the areola were probably what earlier authors referred to as milk sinuses. They are most likely the first branch of the imaged ducts occurring beneath the areola. Because the breast is not static during lactation, the widened ductal areas would further enlarge during milk let down, giving the impression of the presence of milk sinuses. Enlargement of the ducts also occurred at areas where multiple branches of ductwork merged (Ramsey et al., 2005). Gooding, Finlay, Shipley, Halliwell, and Duck (2010) confirmed the absence of "milk sinuses," ampullae, or "saclike" features behind the areola. Their 3D ultrasound scanning showed that the widening of a duct in the nipple generally occurred after the first branching point and that there were no structures behind the areola that could be described as lactiferous sinuses.

Milk Ducts

Milk ducts at the base of the nipple are very superficial and easily compressed. Their depth ranged from 0.7 to 7.9 mm. This anatomic feature bears some watchfulness as excessive compression or compression applied incorrectly may occlude these ducts, impeding the flow of milk out of the nipple. Proper latch and sucking become important for clinicians to monitor as does the fit of the shield or flange on a breast pump to avoid excessive pressure on the superficial ductwork of the nipple. Ducts are not always arranged symmetrically and their course is often erratic.

Using histological cross sections, Taneri and colleagues (2006) studied the number and diameter of milk ducts in the nipple and investigated the possible effects of age, breast weight, and diameter of the nipple on the number of ducts in the nipple duct bundle. There was a positive correlation between number of ducts in the nipple and the size of the nipple, with a range of 8 to 30 ducts found in the nipple. Going and Mohun (2006) used digital modeling of 2 mm sections of breast tissue to describe breast duct branching. The researchers confirmed that some of the ducts within the nipple could be traced to the skin surface, while others could not. No duct branching was seen in the first 2 mm below the skin surface.

Rusby et al. (2007) studied the number of ducts within the nipple and related those to the number of orifices on the nipple surface. They found a mean of 24 ducts within sectioned nipples, with a range of 5–50 ducts. Although Ramsey et al. (2005) found approximately nine ducts in the nipple, it must be remembered that ultrasound cannot identify ducts of less than 0.5 mm. Several ducts can arise from the same cleft in the nipple tip, accounting for the discrepancy between the number of ducts in the nipple and the number of openings that can be counted externally. The shared opening of multiple ducts on the surface of the nipple tip can be seen in **Figure 1-2**.

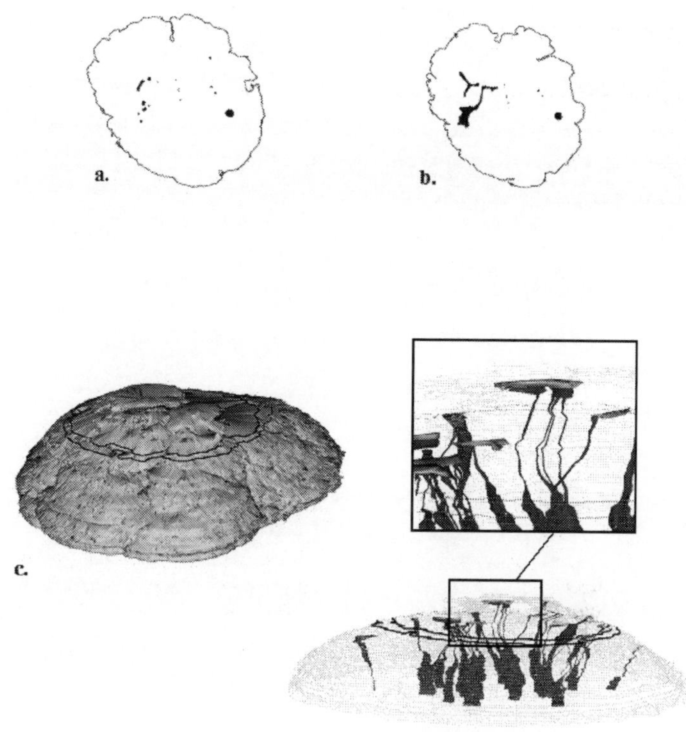

Figure 1-2. Three Dimensional Reconstruction of a Nipple from Sectioned Nipple Specimens

a, b: Two sections of the nipple tip. Many small ducts in upper left quadrant of section a arise from a cleft in section b, 100 micrometers nearer the tip. c, d: Three dimensional reconstruction of a nipple tip.
From (Rusby et al., 2007). Reprinted with kind permission from Springer Science+Business Media.

There is usually a group of central orifices with peripheral ductal openings surrounding the central openings in a somewhat concentric pattern. Most ducts are arranged in a central bundle that narrows to a "waist" approximately 2 mm beneath the skin (**Figure 1-3**).

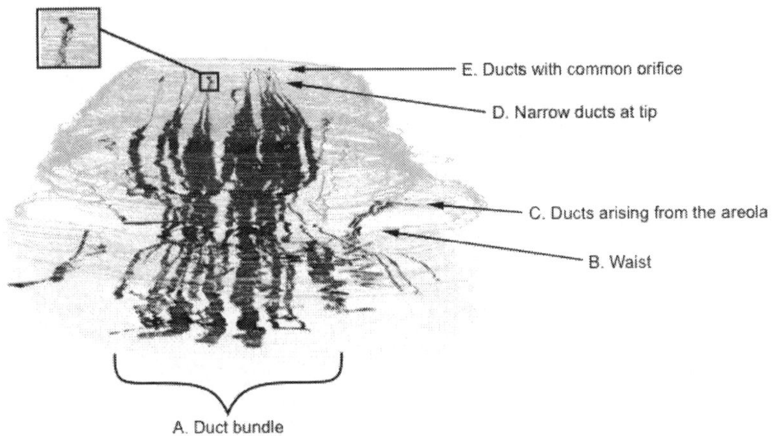

Figure 1-3. Pattern of Ducts within the Nipple

Three-dimensional reconstruction of a nipple. The ducts are arranged in a central bundle, with the bundle narrowing to a waist just beneath the skin. Some ducts originate on the areola or part way up the nipple, with most ducts narrowing as they approach the tip of the nipple. Many of the ducts originate from a few clefts.

From (Rusby et al., 2007). Reprinted with kind permission from Springer Science+Business Media.

This central bundle of ducts occupies 21–67% of the cross-sectional area of the nipple. Multiple ducts may branch and end within the nipple, whereas others end as lobular tissue or as a blind-ending sinus. Other ducts originate at the base of the nipple and on the areola and are morphologically different from the ducts within the central bundle. At 1 and 1.5 mm beneath the tip of the nipple, the average duct diameter is 0.06 mm. However, this increased more than 10-fold to 0.7 mm at a 3 mm depth. There is no relationship between the size of the duct and whether it ended within the nipple or passed deeper into the breast. The other types often disappear into a skin appendage and are most likely tubercles, tubes, sebaceous (oil-secreting) gland orifices, and sweat gland openings that lie superficial to the areola, but do not communicate with the milk-secreting and transporting apparatus. Duct diameters greater than 2–3 mm are considered enlarged and may indicate ductal ectasia (a benign condition of swollen clogged ducts) or mastalgia (unspecified breast pain), but ductal diameters can also range from 0.6 to 4.4 mm with no evidence of pathology (Ballesio et al., 2007; Peters, Diemer, Mecks, & Behnken, 2003; Tedeschi, Ahari, & Byrne, 1963). **Figures 1-2 and 1-3** currently represent the best accounting and "visualization" of the arrangement of the nipple's ductal system.

Nipple Classification

Nipples vary in size and shape, with some variations carrying the potential for a difficult latch, such as those that are flat, inverted, dimpled, bulbous, bifurcated, exceptionally large, or double. Many descriptors have been used to characterize the wide variations in nipples that women present to the breastfeeding experience.

Pseudoinverted Nipple

Pseudoinverted nipples appear inverted, but when the areola around them is compressed, they evert. The connective tissue is thought to be deficient, but the length of the underlying ductwork is normal and an adequately suckling infant will sufficiently elongate the nipple for proper latch (Terrill & Stapleton, 1991).

Inverted Nipple

Failure of the mammary pit to elevate during embryonic development is a result of the lack of mesenchymal proliferation, which pushes the nipple out of its developmentally depressed position (Bland & Romnell, 1991). These are also referred to as tied, invaginated, tethered, or non-protractile (McGeorge, 1994). Inverted nipples seem to be an anatomical fault that has been ascribed to short lactiferous ducts and a fibrous alteration of the subareolar connective tissue that tether the nipple and prevent it from projecting. The retraction caused by the highly resistant collagen fibers in which the lactiferous ducts are embedded can be corrected with surgery, but differing surgical procedures run the risk of severing the lactiferous ducts in the nipple, limiting or preventing milk removal. Definitions of nipple types vary and some of the terms are used interchangeably. Inverted or non-protractile nipples have been reported to occur in 7% to 10% of pregnant women who wish to breastfeed (Alexander, 1992; Hytten & Baird, 1958).

The prevalence of congenital inverted nipples was studied by Park, Yoon, and Kim (1999) in a sample of 1,625 women between the ages of 19 and 26. The anomaly was found in 3.05% of the 3,250 nipples. Fifty-three women presented with the condition. It occurred as bilateral in 46 of the women (86.79%) and unilateral in seven women (13.21%). Of the total number of congenital inverted nipples, 96.23% were umbilicated and 3.77% were invaginated. An inverted nipple is inherited about 50% of the time, and the remaining 50% result from trauma, disease, or surgical procedures.

Plastic surgeons have graded inverted nipples through evaluation and surgical confirmation relative to the degree of fibrosis (replacement of normal cells with connective tissue, similar to scar tissue) (Han & Hong, 1999).

Grade I: The nipple is easily pulled out manually, maintains its protrusion or projection, and contains minimal fibrosis.

Grade II: The nipple can be manually pulled out, but does not maintain its protrusion, retreating back into the areola, and is thought to have moderate fibrosis beneath the nipple.

Grade III: The nipple can barely be manually pulled out, with severe fibrotic bands and less soft tissue underlying the nipple.

In a study of 300 Japanese women (600 breasts), Sanuki, Fukama, and Uchida (2008) measured the diameter of the nipple-areola complex and the height of the nipple. The nipple shapes were classified into four types (**Figure 1-4**).

Type I: when the nipple height was greater than the diameter

Type II: when the nipple height was shorter than the diameter

Type III: when the nipple was inverted

Type IV: when the nipple was of other shapes, such as multiple or divided

They also subclassified types I and II according to the location of strictures. The mean diameter of the nipple was 1.3 cm (range, 0.6–2.3 cm), the mean height of the nipple was 0.9 cm (range, 0–2.0 cm), and the mean diameter of the areola was 4.0 cm (range, 2.0-7.0 cm). Type II without constriction was the most common type of nipple (60.2%), followed by type II with constriction (25.3%). Inverted nipples were found in 3.5% of the breasts.

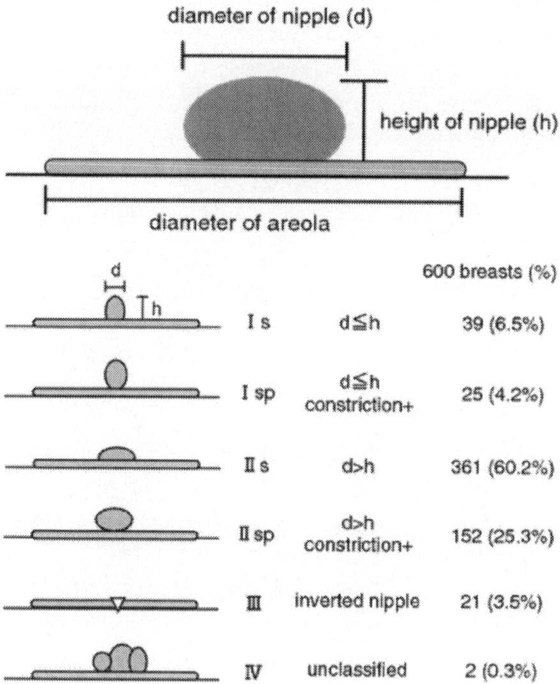

Figure 1-4. Classification Ratio of Nipple Shape

From (Sanuki et al., 2008). Reprinted with kind permission from Springer Science + Business Media.

Other Causes of Nipple Inversion

Inversion or retraction of the nipple may be present for reasons that are not congenital, such as mastitis or surgery. Retraction may also be seen with:

Breast carcinoma: Timing of the onset of nipple retraction is of great importance. Recent nipple retraction has serious implications. It results from scar tissue formation within a lesion or large mammary duct. As the scar tissue shortens, it pulls adjacent tissue inward, causing nipple deviation, flattening, and finally, retraction. Unilateral nipple retraction, even slight, is also more suspicious than bilateral nipple inversion.

Fat necrosis: A benign inflammatory condition in which painless, round, firm lumps caused by damaged and disintegrating fatty tissues form in the breast tissue, which may have nipple retraction as a sign. Fat necrosis often occurs in women with very large breasts or in response to a bruise or blow to the breast. Fat necrosis is most common in obese, usually middle-aged women with fatty, pendulous breasts. The most common causes of fat necrosis are surgery (biopsy, lumpectomy, reduction mammoplasty, implant removal, breast reconstruction) and radiation therapy. Another important cause is trauma, including blunt chest trauma, seat-belt injury, and even minor trauma that the woman may not recollect.

Breast abscesses occasionally produce retraction of the nipple.

Mammary duct ectasia: More common in middle-age women, milk ducts may become swollen and clogged, with the walls thickening to the point where fluid movement is blocked. Duct ectasia can feel like a small lump just under the nipple. The nipple and areola may become tender and irritated, and turn pink or red. Thick, sticky discharge from the nipple can be black, grey, or greenish in color. In some cases, the nipple may retract. This is a benign (non-cancerous) condition.

Flat Nipples

Dewey et al. (2003) reported a 9% incidence of flat or inverted nipples on the day the baby was born and a 7% incidence seven days later. Although flat nipples are usually unable to be visually assessed, some inverted or dimpled nipples are easily seen during the prenatal period. A dimpled nipple folds back in on itself, with moist tissues adhering and setting the stage for skin breakdown after breastfeeding begins. The "pinch test" or compressing the areola can reveal flat or retracted nipples because there is little protrusion and lack of definition between where the nipple ends and the areolar tissue begins. Nipples typically gain elasticity throughout the pregnancy, and the degree of inversion decreases with subsequent pregnancies.

Early data failed to find an association between an infant's ability to breastfeed successfully and the extent of maternal nipple protrusion (Inch, 1989). However, in a review of five infants admitted to the hospital with severe dehydration and hypernatremia, three of the mothers had inverted nipples and had experienced problems with their infants attaining a proper latch (Cooper, Atherton, Kahana, & Kotagal, 1995). Dewey, Nommsen-Rivers, Heinig, and Cohen (2003) showed that suboptimal infant breastfeeding behavior (defined as scoring less than or equal to 10 on the IBFAT breastfeeding assessment tool) and delayed onset of lactation were significantly related to the presence of flat or inverted nipples on days one, three, and seven postpartum. They specifically recommend that women with flat or inverted nipples be given special breastfeeding assistance until the infant is able to latch effectively. Flat nipples can be detected when the areola is compressed and the nipple flattens to the level of the areola or recedes into the areola.

Other Causes of Flat Nipples

The following other causes of flat nipples, besides anatomical or congenital, have been described:

Overweight or obesity. Overweight or obese mothers may experience a flattened areola and nipple due to excess periareolar adipose tissue (Jevitt, Hernandez, & Groer, 2007). The breast is a repository of fat. As excess fat accumulates, it may serve to expand the areola to the point where increased traction is placed on the nipple itself, stretching it at its base with resultant flattening.

Breast or areolar edema. Breast and areolar edema may distort the nipple/areolar complex to the point where the nipple flattens, causing difficulty for some babies in achieving proper latch (Cotterman, 2004; Miller & Riordan, 2004). Nipples flattened by fluid distention in the breast and areola are also at increased risk for pain and damage from the infant's latching attempts or sucking on a distorted nipple. Normal pregnancies are characterized by increased water retention of up to 8.5 liters of fluid. Excessive IV fluids during labor, oxytocin-induced labor, and preeclampsia can further add to the fluid burden. Large amounts of IV fluids during labor and delivery dilutes plasma proteins, resulting in excess interstitial fluid. Vasopressin, the antidiuretic hormone, is naturally elevated during pregnancy and is structurally similar to oxytocin. High-dose oxytocin infusions during inductions, augmentation of labor, or as a postpartum bolus further exacerbate fluid retention.

Renal clearance during preeclampsia is impaired, increasing fluid stores that are retained even after delivery. As excess fluid shifts to different compartments in the body, the areolar compartment may receive its share of excess fluid, swelling and enveloping the nipple. Excessive fluid in the areola impedes the nipple/areolar complex from being easily drawn into the infant's mouth and alters the alignment of the ducts and connective tissue within it.

When ducts within the nipple and areola cannot be drawn into the form of a teat, nipple damage and reduced milk transfer may result. Placing a breast pump on an already edematous areola to pull out the "flat" nipple may further serve to draw more fluid into an already congested area. An areola that demonstrates pitting edema (a pit is formed from fingertip pressure) may contain enough excess fluid to hide even a normally everted nipple. A shiny and taut areola may signal fluid congestion in deeper tissues and be indicative of an edematous process that has continued for an extended period of time.

Dimpled and Retracted Nipples

Dimpled and retracted nipples involve only part of the nipple. A retracted nipple appears as a slit-like area that is pulled inward on the tip of the nipple. A dimpled nipple folds in on itself around part or all of the circumference of the nipple tip. Both types of nipples have the potential for causing problems. Tissue within the slit or dimple may retain significant moisture following breastfeeding or breast pumping. As this tissue folds back and adheres to itself, it may not have the opportunity to dry. This presents the conditions for the nipples to become macerated and serves as a breeding ground for bacteria and fungal overgrowth. Dimpled and retracted nipples may be either unilateral or bilateral.

Double or Bifurcated Nipples

The occurrence of double or bifurcated nipples is termed intra-areolar polythelia (**Figure 1-5**) and is often hereditary (Abramson, 1975). Two or more supernumerary nipples are located within the areola, which is believed to be caused by intrauterine division of the embryonic breast or nipple (Abramson, 1975). Each nipple may have its own ductal system (Onesti, Anniboletti, Spinelli, & Meggiorini, 2008), with multiple nipples located on one or both areolae. The areolar diameter may be enlarged on the affected side to the point of being double the size of the unaffected areola (Lopez, Garcia, Elena, Benito, & Juan, 2006). The multiple nipples may be completely separate from each other or may be joined by a ridge of areolar tissue.

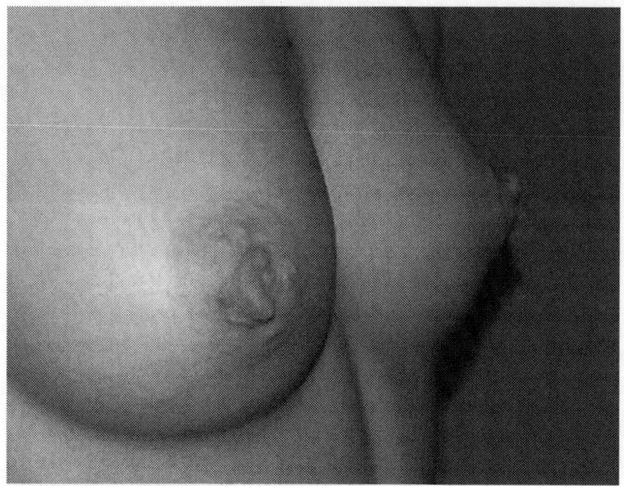

Figure 1-5. Bilateral Intra-Areolar Polythelia (two nipples on each breast)
From (Onesti et al., 2008). Reprinted with kind permission from Springer Science+Business Media.

Breastfeeding is usually quite possible from unusually presenting nipples (Lopez, Sorando, Martinez, & Bravo, 2005; Baratelli & Vischi, 1999). Mothers may need to position the infant such that both nipples can be effectively drawn into the infant's mouth without pain or damage to either nipple. Some arrangements of bifurcated nipples present as a cluster of "nipples" resembling a mulberry. If this cluster is very large, the infant may have difficulty drawing the entire structure into his mouth. If the breast is to be pumped, care must be taken in the selection of a properly sized flange. The double nipple or the entire arrangement of nipples must fit comfortably into the flange tunnel to avoid pain and tissue damage and to extract optimal amounts of milk.

PHYSIOLOGY OF THE NIPPLE DURING SUCKING

Infant sucking has long been of interest to researchers and healthcare providers. Prior to the sophisticated imaging equipment currently in use, descriptions from visual observations of infants at breast were used to speculate on infant sucking mechanisms and the behavior of the breast inside the infant's mouth. Researchers have provided varying descriptions (see below) of the nipple and what forces were exerted and responsible for milk transfer. Some observations were remarkably similar to current reports, while others contributed to the long-held belief that milk was extracted from the breast either from the jaws clamping down on milk ducts lying beneath the areola or from a stripping action of the tongue beneath the nipple. The currently held view of the sucking mechanism and the action of the nipple within the infant's mouth is described in the Geddes et al. (2008a) summary.

- **Emslie (1931):** Emslie described the sucking mechanism as a rhythmical clamping of the jaws that compressed and relaxed ampullae (milk sinuses) in the areola, pushing milk forward into the infant's mouth where suction ultimately withdrew the milk.
- **Waller (1938, 1943, 1947):** Waller subscribed to the view that milk was obtained by compression of the milk sinuses between the jaws. He believed that suction was used only to draw the nipple into the mouth.
- **Evans & MacKeith (1954):** Evans and MacKeith likened the nipple to a cherry on a stalk. They described the nipple as being held well back in the mouth by suction, with the gums closing on the areola, the tongue pressing the nipple and areola against the hard palate, and the milk being expressed partly by compression of the milk cisterns (sinuses) and partly by suction.
- **Ardran and Kemp (1958):** Ardran and Kemp were some of the first researchers to visualize the breast inside the infant's mouth. In their study, the breast was coated with a barium sulfate paste, and radiographic films were made while the infant nursed. Infants were positioned lying down on a couch with the mother leaning over the baby, which may have prevented a deep latch and partially accounted for observations that have since been refined with newer imaging techniques. Notable was the confirmation that the nipple and areola were drawn into the mouth close to the junction of the

hard and soft palates and that the nipple widened and extended to about three times its resting length, forming the nipple–areolar complex or a teat. These authors also described the action of the infant forming the nipple–areola into a teat and drawing it far back into the mouth, with the tongue playing a major part in the sucking process and the breast being soft and pliable enough to allow this activity. According to these authors, "Any factor which causes edema or congestion [of the breast] will probably interfere with suckling."

- They stated that sucking at the breast was similar to bottle feeding, as the tongue compressed the nipple/areolar complex against the palate and indented the nipple, with the tongue action moving from front to back. The contents of the ducts were compressed and expressed into the mouth by a stripping action. They believed that milk expression occurred due to compression of the nipple between the tongue and palate. They could not describe what the action of suction was responsible for other than drawing the nipple into the mouth. Their study was confined to the lateral plane and could not visualize other tongue actions. It also relied on x-rays, whose hazards halted the use of this type of research.
- **Smith and colleagues (1985):** Smith, Erenberg, Nowak, and Franken studied 16 breastfed infants using real-time ultrasound. They reported that failure of the lips to form a complete seal was seen on the ultrasound scan as air leaking into the oral cavity. The buccal mucosa and musculature (sucking pads, buccinator muscle) moved inward as the tongue was depressed. This maintained a tight seal on the nipple–areola. The tongue was seen to form a depression or groove in its posterior portion which conducted the milk toward the oropharynx, with the nipple elongated during active sucking and then retracting at a rapid rate after the milk was expressed.
- **Weber and colleagues (1986):** Weber, Woolridge, and Baum studied infants under ultrasound and described that during a suck cycle, the action of the tongue appeared as a rolling or peristaltic undulation in an anterior to posterior direction, whereas in bottle-fed infants the tongue worked in an up-and-down piston-type motion. When not sucking, the breastfed infants maintained their grasp on the nipple, with the teat still moderately indented by the tongue.
- **Woolridge (1986a):** Woolridge described a suck cycle as the infant exerting suction to draw the nipple and part of the areola into the

mouth, with the nipple extending three times its resting length to the junction of the hard and soft palate. Milk was thought to be expressed from the ampullae (milk sinuses) under the nipple/areola and propelled to the back of the mouth by a peristaltic wave-like motion of the tongue. The roller-like action of the tongue was stated to squeeze milk from the nipple as the wave of tongue compression moved backwards. The lowering of the jaw was described as allowing milk to flow back into the nipple (not as the mechanism for the release of milk from the nipple). Compression was thought to be the primary driving force of milk movement out of the nipple. The nipple occupied as much space in the infant's mouth as there was nipple/areolar tissue to fill it. The shape of the nipple within the mouth was described as being dictated by the internal geometry of the mouth, with no free space surrounding it. **Figure 1-6** depicts a graphic representation of the suck cycle according to Woolridge and has been used in numerous lactation texts as descriptive of the typical mechanics of milk removal from the breast.

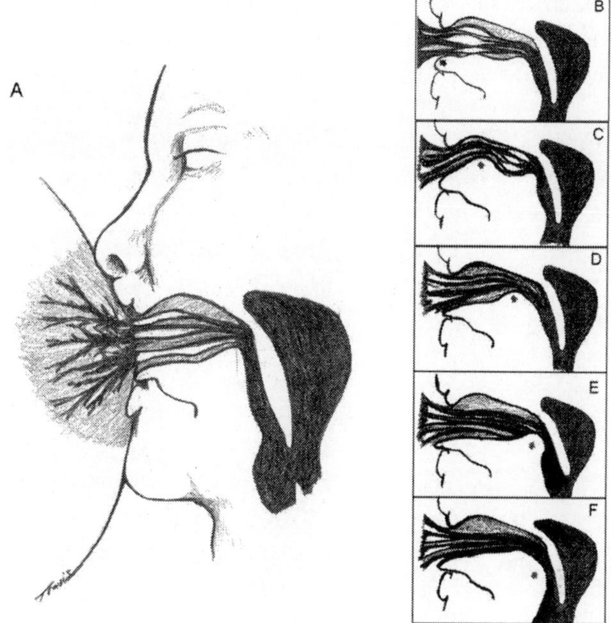

Complete suck cycle. The baby is shown in median section.
The baby exhibits good feeding technique: the nipple is drawn well into the mouth, extending back to the junction of the hard and soft palate (the lactiferous sinuses are depicted within the teat, although these cannot be visualized on scans).

Figure 1-6. Complete Suck Cycle Under Ultrasound
From (Woolridge, 1986a). Reprinted with permission from Elsevier.

- **Smith and colleagues (1988):** Smith, Erenberg, and Nowak imaged 16 term breastfeeding infants using real-time ultrasound. They reported that the nipple was highly elastic, elongating to twice its resting length, and at maximal compression, nipple height was reduced by half. Infants were described as using an up-and-down piston-like movement of the mandible, tongue, and hyoid, rather than an undulant or peristaltic movement. They correctly reported that peristaltic tongue movement did not cause milk to be ejected from the nipple. Milk ejection occurred 0.03 seconds after maximal nipple deformation and coincided with the dropping of the tongue and jaw. The jaw actually created the negative pressure by enlarging the oral cavity and acted as the stimulus for the release of milk from the nipple. Their data suggested that nipple compression may draw milk into the nipple ducts, but the actual mechanism for milk ejection was the formation of a vacuum when the jaw and tongue lowered.

Currently, more sensitive ultrasound studies have allowed a better visualization of the nipple within the infant's mouth and have provided a clearer description of nipple positioning and sucking dynamics. The following 2 studies offer the most current explanation of the behavior of the nipple in the infant's mouth and the factors contributing to the release of milk from the nipple.

- **Jacobs and colleagues (2007):** Nipple position within the infant's mouth is an important factor in the effective and pain-free transfer of milk from the breast to the infant. Jacobs and colleagues utilized submental ultrasound images to measure the distance from the tip of the nipple to the junction of the hard and soft palate in 18 mother/baby pairs during the first and fourth weeks of life. Many depictions of nipple positioning within the mouth show the nipple tip located at the junction of the hard and soft palate when fully elongated.

  Nipple position and its relationship to the hard and soft palate junction had not actually been measured until Jacobs and colleagues studied this facet of breastfeeding. Their measurements revealed that the median distance from the tip of the nipple to the junction of the hard and soft palates was 5 mm in both weeks one and four, with a range of 2.7 to 9.9 mm in week one and 3.2 to 8.7 mm in week four. However, sucking is a dynamic process and measurement of nipple positioning at a single moment in time is important, but must also be considered within the total suck cycle. There was a range of nipple movement during the suck cycle, which had a mean of 4 mm. Excessive nipple movement or movement beyond these parameters may contribute to sucking problems and sore nipples.

  Only 25% of the infants in this study drew the nipple to the point of the hard and soft palate junction. The nipple remained 5 mm anterior to the hard and soft palate junction in 50% of the infants. During slow-motion videotapes, this study also revealed that when the tongue was in its most upright position holding the nipple against the hard palate, no milk was compressed into the mouth. When the tongue moved downward and posterior to the nipple tip, milk was seen being released from the nipple.

- **Geddes and colleagues (2008a):** Geddes and colleagues used ultrasound to observe movements of the tongue during breastfeeding in 20 breastfed infants and relate these movements to milk flow and intra-oral vacuum (**Figure 1**-7). Their findings are summarized below.

First, negative pressure draws the nipple–areola into the mouth, usually several millimeters anterior to the junction of the hard and soft palate forming a teat. A baseline vacuum of -64 + 45 mm Hg is maintained over the entire feeding. The baseline vacuum is a result of the seal formed by the lips and the downward movement of the jaw when the infant first latches to the breast. Baseline vacuums may be difficult for some infants to maintain, such as preterm infants or those with neurological conditions, as evidenced by slippage off of the breast, a shallow latch, sore nipples, or ineffective milk transfer.

Second, the motion of the tongue during a suck cycle does not show a peristaltic action (as in bottle-feeding), but rather the tongue is up at the start of a suck cycle and in apposition with the hard palate, with the anterior tongue not indenting the nipple. Vacuum is generated as the tongue and jaw move down, which allows milk to flow from the nipple and the nipple ducts to become visible on ultrasound. Peak vacuum coincides with the tongue at its lowermost position.

As the tongue moves back up, vacuum decreases and milk flow ceases. The tongue captures the milk that has flowed into the nipple, holding it in place until the tongue and jaw lower again, with the milk subsequently flowing into the oral cavity. This mechanism ensures that milk is not constantly flowing into the oral cavity, but is apportioned into manageable boluses, so that excessive swallowing does not interfere with breathing and oxygenation. Nipple diameter was greater when the tongue was in the down position, and the distance from the tip of the nipple to the junction of the hard and soft palate was greater when the tongue was in the up position.

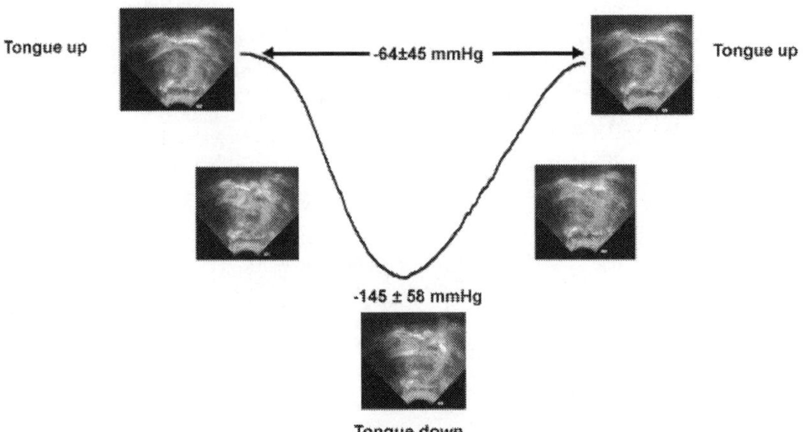

Figure 1-7. Changes in Infant Tongue Position During One Suck Cycle
From (Geddes et al., 2008a). Reprinted with permission from Elsevier.

Vacuum was shown to be the primary force in milk removal, rather than a stripping action of the tongue. Neither milk flow nor milk ducts were observed in the nipple when the tongue was squeezing the nipple. During vacuum generation as the tongue lowered, the nipple expanded, allowing the ducts within the nipple to be visible on ultrasound, and the nipple moved closer to the junction of the hard and soft palate.

Section 2

Nipple Problems and Their Management

Nipple problems in lactating mothers have been mentioned in the medical literature since the 1500s (Fildes, 1986). Breastfeeding aids designed to remedy inverted and/or sore nipples are described in these early medical texts. Sucking glasses were used to evert flat nipples. Nipple shields made from wood, pewter, lead, tin, ivory, silver, or glass were used to evert nipples or to place over sore nipples while the infant breastfed.

Mothers still experience these nipple problems today. Nipple variations can contribute to poor breastfeeding outcomes, including poor or ineffective milk transfer, poor infant sucking skills, delayed lactogenesis II, and excess newborn weight loss (Dewey et al., 2003; Vazirinejad, Darakhshan, Esmaeili, & Hadadian, 2009). Clinicians work to prevent or remedy a plethora of problems related either to the anatomy and physiology of the nipple or to the sucking dynamics that each infant brings to the experience.

ANTENATAL NIPPLE PREPARATION

Methods of antenatal nipple conditioning were taught to women for decades in the belief that prenatal preparation would correct nipple defects and prevent sore nipples (Cadwell, 1981; Otte, 1975). Most of these rituals have been abandoned, as research has yet to confirm that antenatal preparation causes the desired changes in nipple structure and/or results in pain-free outcomes.

Nipple Rolling

Applebaum (1969) believed that antenatal stretching of the nipple was important if it was flat or inverted, as this procedure would cause it to be more elastic and less likely to retract. Nipple rolling involved pulling out the nipple to its outermost position and either holding it or rolling it. This was repeated 10 times twice a day to increase elasticity of the tissue. However, subsequent research indicated that this was not consistently an effective strategy for reducing nipple soreness. For example, Whitley (1978) used a 68-item questionnaire in a telephone survey and found that prenatal nipple rolling did not prevent sore nipples. Sixty-seven percent of the subjects who prepared their nipples and 50% of those that did not experienced sore nipples postpartum.

Similarly, Brown and Hurlock (1975) evaluated the effectiveness of three prenatal nipple preparation techniques: nipple rolling, application of

Masse Cream, and prenatal expression of colostrum in 57 women. Each woman conditioned one nipple, but not the other, for approximately three weeks prior to delivery, serving as her own control. Following delivery, subjective and objective observations revealed that there were no significant differences in either subjective or objective measures of nipple sensitivity or trauma in any of the three groups. The researchers concluded that these methods of nipple preparation were ineffective.

In another study, 17 women conditioned one of their nipples for six weeks before their expected delivery date (Atkinson, 1979). One nipple was rolled twice a day for two minutes, rubbed for 15 seconds once a day with a terry cloth towel, and aired for two hours each day with the outer clothing allowed to rub against the nipple. Each woman served as her own control. The nipple conditioning was shown to significantly reduce the amount of total nipple pain experienced on the conditioned nipple during the first few days of breastfeeding. Fair-skinned women in this study reported more nipple soreness on the unconditioned nipple. No mention was made regarding whether measures were taken in the hospital to observe if the baby was positioned and latched correctly as the contributor to sore nipples.

Fleming (1984) partially replicated Atkinson's study by having 17 mothers start conditioning their nipples six weeks prior to delivery by rubbing one nipple with a terry cloth towel 15 seconds daily, nipple rolling for two minutes twice daily, and airing the nipple so it would rub against the outer clothing for two hours a day. The nipples that had been conditioned were reported to have no or slight soreness that disappeared shortly after the infant began to suck, while the unconditioned nipples were reported more often as experiencing extreme pain that continued throughout the nursing period. No mention was made regarding whether measures were taken in the hospital to observe if the baby was positioned and latched correctly as the contributor to sore nipples.

In a study with similar methodology (Storr, 1988), 25 women served as their own controls by preparing one nipple for six weeks prior to delivery, using nipple rolling twice daily for 30 seconds and rubbing the nipple gently with a terry towel for 15 seconds twice daily. Mothers reported significantly less pain on the prepared nipple than on the unconditioned nipple. Remedial methods of addressing nipple pain in the hospital were not studied.

Hoffman's Exercises

Hoffman (1953) thought that flat nipples were anchored to the areola by adhesions at their base. He recommended a procedure in which the thumbs or index fingers were positioned on each side of the nipple and the areola was stretched sideways 5 times, and then stretched in the vertical plane five times, a couple of times each day. Traction at the base of the nipple was believed to eventually loosen or break adhesions and allow the nipple to move more freely.

In the MAIN trial collaborative group (1994), 442 mothers were randomized into four groups and asked to prepare their nipples using either Hoffman's exercises five times twice per day, wearing breast shells through the daytime, or using both breast shells and Hoffman's exercise, with the last group engaged in no preparation of their nipples during pregnancy. Results showed no evidence that either Hoffman's exercises or breast shells or both would increase the likelihood of mothers breastfeeding at six weeks after birth. Based on the Alexander (1992) study and the MAIN study, Hoffman's exercises and the wearing of breast shells fell out of favor with clinicians and are seldom recommended anymore.

Breast Shells

Breast shells (also called Woolwich Shields, Netsy Cups, Hobbit Shells, Swedish Milk Cups) are a two-piece system consisting of a flat disk with a hole in the center through which the nipple protrudes. The disk is covered by a vented dome and placed under the bra to exert pressure on the base of the nipple "to gradually stretch and loosen its attachment to the deep structures of the breast" (Waller, 1946).

Waller (1946) recommended wearing breast shells during the daytime for the last three months of the pregnancy. The early breast shells were made of glass and were originally used during the Victorian era to collect leaking milk and protect clothing. To determine whether wearing breast shells prenatally was necessary, Waller recommended doing the "pinch test" by squeezing the areola just beyond the base of the nipple to see if it would flatten or retract. This action was thought to mimic the action of the baby at breast and show what the nipple would do in the infant's mouth during latch. If the nipple flattened, it was believed to be too firmly attached to deep structures within the areola.

Alexander, Grant, and Campbell (1992) randomized 96 subjects into four possible prenatal treatment options: breast shells alone, Hoffman's exercises alone, both breast shells and Hoffman's exercises, and no preparation. Results of this randomized controlled trial of breast shells and Hoffman's exercises showed that there was little difference among the groups in sustained improvement in nipple anatomy and that fewer mothers who used breast shells were breastfeeding six weeks after delivery.

Mechanical Stretching of the Nipple by Suction

Gangal and Gangal (1978) wrote of the Gangal aspirator to mechanically pull out inverted nipples. A device called the Niplette (Avent) uses the concept of tissue expansion through continuous long-term suction, derived from the disciplines of plastic and aesthetic surgery. McGeorge (1994) thought that short lactiferous ducts tethered the nipple, which prevented it from projecting. This device consists of a transparent thimble-like nipple mold with a syringe port. The mold is placed over the flat nipple, air is evacuated from the mold by the connected syringe, and the nipple is slowly drawn out to the mother's comfort and held in place while the device is worn.

The device is worn eight or more hours a day during the first six months of the pregnancy. The Niplette has a tendency to fall off, so mothers are advised to place a small amount of Vaseline or other lubricant around the base of the mold to improve the seal. Successful breastfeeding has been reported in a small number of mothers with the use of the device, but it has the potential for pain and nipple bleeding if too much suction is applied. It can be used briefly before each feeding in the first few days post birth, but the presence of milk in the mold impairs the device's suction.

Nipple Rubbing

Nipple rubbing was often recommended prenatally, as it was thought that friction from a towel rubbing against the nipples each day would build a thicker or stronger keratin layer over the nipple. This extra layer was supposed to protect the nipple from the action of the infant's tongue during breastfeeding. Newton (1952) observed that mothers with four or more children reported less nipple pain and damage than first-time mothers or mothers with fewer children. She extrapolated from this observation that it might be useful for mothers to simulate use of the nipples before the birth of the infant to reduce nipple pain when breastfeeding. She suggested that this could be done by holding the nipple in a rough towel and pulling outwards several times.

Zeimer and colleagues (1990) conducted a study on 100 breastfeeding mothers to evaluate nipple pain in the early postpartum period. Of the

100 mothers in the study, 96 reported nipple pain at some time during the six-week study. Of the sample, 65% had engaged in some form of prenatal nipple preparation that included methods such as nipple rolling, rubbing with a terry towel, applying creams or ointments, going braless, and avoiding the use of soap on the nipples. Nipple pain developed in many of these mothers in spite of prenatal efforts to prevent it.

Avoiding the Use of Soap on the Nipples

Newton (1952) found that mothers in her study who were instructed to wash their nipples with a soap solution prior to feeding their infant experienced a high incidence of nipple pain and nipple damage. The particular soap solution had additives of a detergent and a chelating agent that rendered it more potent and more destructive to the nipple epidermis. Newton stated that even pure soap would weaken the nipple skin and recommended that one step in the prevention of nipple pain and damage was to instruct pregnant and lactating women to avoid the use of soap on the nipples. No further studies could be found to support this conjecture, and women have been told to this day to avoid using soap on their nipples in spite of little supporting evidence.

Surgery for Truly Inverted Nipples

Surgery to correct inverted nipples has long been practiced, mostly as a cosmetic procedure. Surgery on the nipple, however, has a high potential for damaging or destroying the tiny ducts within the nipple. Ducts can be spared by surgery that is meant only to release fibrous adhesions between ducts that may be exerting traction on the nipple. Cutting these restricting ducts would evert the nipple, but significantly increase the chance of problems with milk flow from that breast.

Evaluation of Effectiveness of Prenatal Preparation

A number of researchers have studied and compared prenatal preparation techniques to establish which ones were more effective. In general, most of the results are inconclusive or mixed, with few, if any, definitive studies or recommendations. Almost all prenatal nipple preparation techniques have been abandoned due to lack of high-quality evidence that any of them contribute to a reduction in nipple soreness. Some mothers with severely inverted nipples use the Niplette to mechanically stretch the internal anchoring tissues. Mothers with dry, peeling nipple and areolar skin may wish to use an emollient to avoid beginning breastfeeding with nipple and areolar skin that is already damaged or at increased risk for early breakdown. Any pre-existing nipple/areolar skin conditions, such as eczema, psoriasis, etc., should be remedied prior to the infant's birth.

FLAT AND INVERTED NIPPLES

Flat nipples may not be apparent either in the prenatal period or in the intrapartum period until the infant demonstrates latching difficulty or the nipples become sore or damaged. Waller (1946) described the potential problems of a flat nipple in that it would fail to be drawn far enough into the infant's mouth and would be subject to frictional forces that could break the skin integrity and place the milk ducts within the nipple in an unphysiological position. He recommended that a simple test be performed in the prenatal period to simulate the action of the nipple/areola when grasped by the infant. This came to be popularly known as the "pinch test" and was done by compressing the areola between the thumb and index finger approximately ¼ to ½ inch beyond where the nipple joins the areola. This simulation would cause a flat nipple to pull back either flush or almost flush with the areolar skin and an inverted nipple to retract below the level of the areola. This procedure became a routine part of prenatal breastfeeding education for decades. This, along with other preparation techniques, was for the most part abandoned, as it was thought that complicated or time-consuming preparation procedures would discourage women from breastfeeding.

Dewey and colleagues (2003) conducted a study to determine the incidence of and risk factors for suboptimal breastfeeding behavior, delayed onset of lactogenesis II, and excess newborn weight loss in 280 mother/baby pairs. Suboptimal infant breastfeeding behaviors on the first, third, and seventh day of life were significantly associated with a mother who had flat or inverted nipples. Delayed onset of lactation (>72 hours postpartum) was significantly associated with flat or inverted nipples, as was excess infant weight loss. This is not surprising since effective breastfeeding on the part of the infant depends on the mechanical ability of the infant to form a teat from the nipple and part of the areola and draw it well into the mouth. The authors recommended that a mother with flat or inverted nipples should receive special assistance until the infant is able to latch and feed effectively. Anatomical variations of the nipple that impede this process can contribute not only to delayed lactogenesis II, poor milk transfer, and newborn weight loss, but also to sore nipples, engorgement, and reduced milk production.

Vazirinejad and colleagues (2009) studied 100 primiparous mothers and their neonates. One group of 50 had flat, inverted, or large nipples or large breasts, the other group of 50 did not have these anatomical variations. When infant weights were measured on day seven, the mean weight of neonates who were born to mothers with at least one of the anatomical variations was less than their birth weight. The mean weight of infants on day seven born to mothers without any of these variations was above birth weight and significantly higher than the weight of infants of mothers with nipple variations. The authors recommended that nipple and breast evaluation occur prenatally and routinely on the maternity unit following the birth.

Even though flat and inverted nipples are considered "common" problems and do not attract the attention of clinicians as much as other more hot-button problems, this anatomical variation has the potential to derail breastfeeding right from the start, increasing the chance for formula supplementation, reducing exclusive breastfeeding, and resulting in early weaning. A quick check of the nipples in the prenatal and early postpartum period may help guide the clinician's approach to the best and most effective breastfeeding recommendations for each mother/baby pair.

After the infant has been born is when some urgency arises if the infant cannot latch or transfer milk or if the mother's nipples become sore or damaged. If the nipple does not protrude, the infant does not experience tactile feedback during latch-on that would be given by a firm, everted nipple. Non-protractile, surrounding areolar tissue further impedes latch in some infants. A number of interventions have been suggested to remedy this situation. To help shape the nipple before the infant latches, the mother can place a cold compress on the nipple, gently pull and roll it prior to feedings, or place her thumb and index finger above and below the nipple, pressing inward and together to help "pop" out the nipple.

The flat or inverted nipple can be temporarily everted prior to each feeding such that enough nipple/areolar tissue is presented to the infant to enable the infant to latch. The application of a breast pump has been recommended and used for this purpose. However, a pump distributes vacuum over a relatively large area and has the potential to increase interstitial fluid pressure (Cotterman, 2004), causing nipple swelling (Wilson-Clay & Hoover, 2008). Such swelling creates another layer of fluid within the areola under the area of the pump flange that thickens the superficial areolar tissue and further impedes the infant's ability to latch (Cotterman, 2003). In addition, a pump does not provide a steady, uninterrupted vacuum or a method to control how long and how strongly the vacuum is applied (Kesaree, 1993).

Some mothers find that wearing breast shells under their bra between feedings everts flat nipples. This may result from the displacement of fluid from the continuous pressure exerted by the rim of the nipple opening. However, when the shells are worn for prolonged periods of time and there is significant areolar edema, potential for exacerbating edema and damaging underlying tissues exists from the strangulation of capillary circulation.

A simple and inexpensive tool can be fashioned from a 10 mL disposable plastic syringe. Kesaree, Banapurmath, Banapurmath, and Shamanur (1993) modified the syringe by removing the plunger, cutting off the end of the syringe ¼ inch above where a needle would attach, and inserting the plunger through the end that was cut. The mother then places the smooth end of the syringe directly over her nipple and pulls back gently on the plunger to her comfort for 30 seconds to a minute prior to each feeding. This allows the nipple to be drawn out from the surrounding areola (Thorley, 1997). She should also repeat this procedure several times each day between feedings to more quickly improve nipple protrusion. If the flat nipples persist at discharge, the mother can be instructed to use the device at home until the infant can easily latch to the breast and transfer milk.

Some hospitals prohibit the use of devices which are not FDA approved. Commercial, FDA approved versions of this device are available: the Evert-It Nipple Enhancer (Maternal Concepts) and LatchAssist (Lansinoh). No data are available regarding the effectiveness of these devices and consumer reviews have been mixed.

Other Causes of Flat Nipples

Some nipples may appear flat but are actually enveloped by an edematous areola following labor and delivery. These nipples are not flat, just difficult to access. Large amounts of IV fluids, use of pitocin, or excessive water retention, such as in preeclampsia (Cotterman, 2004; Miller & Riordan, 2004), may contribute to an areola that is so swollen it obliterates the nipple, erasing the definition or boundary between the nipple itself and the external areola. This may remove the normally expected tactile stimulation that the infant's sensitive lips seek at latch-on, leading to a difficult or painful latching process. Cold compresses, cabbage leaves, and foods with a diuretic effect (watermelon) have all been anecdotally recommended to help decrease the swelling.

Areolar Compression and Reverse Pressure Softening

Areolar compression can be done prior to latch attempts on an edematous areola (Miller & Riordan, 2004). The mother applies pressure with both thumbs and index fingers into the areola directly behind the nipple. Indentations are created as interstitial fluid is displaced and the fingers are then placed above and below the initial indentations, working their way up to the margins of the areola. The mother rotates her fingers to a new position behind the nipple and works her way to the outer margin of the areola again until the nipple becomes pliable and easily everted, at which point the baby is brought to the breast.

Reverse pressure softening has a number of variations (Cotterman, 2004) which use the mother's fingertips to create pits around the circumference of the nipple. The mother uses three or four fingertips of each hand to encircle the base of the nipple and push inward for one to three minutes with enough pressure to form six to eight pits. This exposes the nipple and presents a better tactile stimulus for latching. A nipple shield can be applied before or after areolar compression or reverse pressure softening if there appears to be no other way to affect the latch.

Both areolar compression and reverse pressure softening may have an added benefit, which is the stimulation of the milk-ejection reflex. Compression directly on the center or core of the areola at the base of the nipple can have the effect of triggering milk letdown within a minute or two, either from stimulation of the nerves converging in the center of the areola or as a reflex contraction of the myoepithelial cells caused by the pressure alone (Cotterman, 2004).

The "teacup" hold may be tried with a non-engorged breast and non-edematous areola. This involves shaping the nipple/areolar complex into a wedge whose long axis matches the long axis of the open mouth of the baby. The mother or clinician uses a thumb and index finger to grasp the areola directly above the nipple, plus some of the breast tissue above it, and forms as much tissue as possible into a wedge, placing it as deep as possible into the infant's mouth. It is held in place until the infant is latched correctly and sucking well (Wilson-Clay & Hoover, 2008).

Dimpled Nipples

A mother with a dimpled nipple (whose margins fold inward) may experience pain or bleeding when the infant first nurses or a breast pump is applied. The vacuum may pull apart these tissues creating a sensitive area that easily becomes macerated. Once the infant is finished with a feeding or a mother is finished pumping, this type of nipple rapidly folds back in on itself, maintaining a moist environment with a damaged epidermis that can quickly become a site for bacterial and/or fungal infection. It is important that after each feeding the mother keeps these tissues from adhering to each other by placing the nipple in a position that prevents the nipple from reverting to its dimpled configuration. A Velcro dimple ring is a small thin strip of Velcro that attaches to and surrounds the base and shank of the nipple, holding the margins of the nipple tip apart until they have air dried.

Nipple Shields

While breastfeeding and the use of breast pumps and other devices and techniques will help evert flat and inverted nipples over time, some infants are still unable to latch effectively to these types of nipples, but nevertheless must be fed during the time of nipple remediation. Nipple shields can be used to provide tactile feedback and keep the baby feeding at the breast until the nipples are protrusive enough or the infant is skilled enough to effectively latch and feed directly from the anomalous nipple. The use of nipple shields can be quite helpful as an intervention in certain breastfeeding situations (Brigham, 1996; Wilson-Clay, 2003). An understanding of what shields can and cannot accomplish is essential in the clinical decision-making process.

Shields can:

- Therapeutically supply oral stimulation that an infant cannot obtain from the mother's nipples due to inability to latch or transfer milk.
- Create a nipple shape in the infant's mouth if the nipple is flat or inverted.
- Allow extraction of milk by expression with minimal suction, with negative pressure inside the shield tip keeping milk available.
- Draw out a flat or inverted nipple.
- Compensate for weak infant suction.
- Present a stable nipple shape that remains during pauses in sucking bursts.
- Maintain the nipple in a protruded position.

- Affect the rate of milk flow.

Shields cannot:

- Correct milk transfer problems or weight gain if the mother has inadequate milk volume.
- Fix damaged nipples if the cause is not discovered and remedied.
- Replace skilled intervention and close follow-up.

Shield use facilitates learning to feed at the breast, allows supplementation to occur at breast if needed (i.e., thread tubing under or alongside of the shield), encourages nipple protractility, does not overwhelm the mother with gadgets, and avoids the infant fighting at the breast. Shields can also stop a cycle of continuing damage to the nipple, allowing healing to take place while nipple protrusion is improving. Shield use may prevent premature termination of breastfeeding. Use of shields does not affect maternal prolactin levels, and infants are able to gain weight appropriately while using a nipple shield (Chertok, Schneider, & Blackburn, 2006).

The clinician must also consider some of the disadvantages of nipple shield use. These problems were seen more frequently with old-style, thick nipple shields. Currently used shields are manufactured from ultra thin silicone, allowing tactile input to the nerves of the nipple/areola complex. Shields should not used as a substitute for skilled care. Shields may exacerbate the original problem; may lead to insufficient milk volume, inadequate weight gain, or weaning; can be problematic without follow-up; can pinch the nipple and areola, causing abrasion, pain, skin breakdown, and internal trauma to the breast if not applied properly; may result in an infant who will not feed at breast without the shield in place; might predispose the nipple to damage when the infant is put to breast without the shield because the infant may chew rather than suckle; and, unfortunately, might be discarded as a useful intervention in selected situations.

Shields composed of all rubber are no longer seen today. Standard bottle nipples placed over the mother's nipple or attached to a glass or plastic base are not appropriate interventions. Latex and silicone shields are extremely thin and flexible, with a firmer nipple portion. Because the silicone is so thin, more stimulation reaches the areola, and milk volume is not depleted as with the earlier designs. With the increasing reports of latex allergy in the general population, latex-containing shields should be avoided. Silicone shields are available in a number of sizes.

Few data exist in the literature regarding shield selection and instructions for their use (**Box 2-1**). The height of the nipple portion of the shield should not exceed the length of the infant's mouth from the juncture of the hard and soft palates to lip closure (Wilson-Clay & Hoover, 2008). If the height of the teat of a shield is greater than this length, the infant's jaw closure and tongue compression will fall on the shaft of the teat and not over the breast. As many infants do not draw the maternal nipple to the juncture of the hard and soft palate, teat height should be closely checked. The teat must be large enough to allow for the expansion of the nipple during sucking. If the height of the teat is too short for the nipple, it may abrade against the inside of the teat or extrude through the teat holes. The base diameter should fit the mother's nipple, with better results occurring with the shortest teat height and smallest base diameter. Teat heights vary by manufacturer and are available in 16 mm, 20 mm, and 24 mm sizes.

There is no set time to wean an infant (or mother) from shield use. Extended use of the ultrathin silicone shield has not been shown to be detrimental (Bodley & Powers, 1996). Mothers start the shield-weaning process by encouraging skin-to-skin contact next to the nipple, starting the feed with the shield and then removing it, and gradually trying feeds without the shield. The tip of the shield should not be cut off in an attempt to present less and less of the device to the infant. Rough edges may scrape the infant's mouth, and the altered shape and consistency of the shield may not be appropriate to the desired outcome.

Box 2-1. Instructions for Shield

- Choose an appropriate size shield.
- Drip expressed milk onto the outside of the teat to encourage the infant to latch.
- Warm the shield to help it stick.
- Apply the shield (may moisten the edges to help it adhere better) by turning it almost inside out.
- Hand express a little milk into the teat if necessary.
- Use a periodontal syringe to pre-fill the teat if the mother is unable to express colostrum or milk into the teat.
- Use alternate massage to help drain the breast.
- Place tubing inside or outside of the shield for supplementation.
- Check the infant's latch with the shield: The mouth must not close on the shaft of the teat.
- Check that the infant is not just sucking on the tip of the teat.
- Have extra shields on hand as spares.
- Pump after each feeding it trying to boost milk supply.
- Carefully check breasts for plugged ducts and areas that are not draining well.
- Boil shield if yeast is present on the areola; otherwise, the shield should be washed in hot soapy water after each use, rinsed thoroughly, and air dried.
- Perform an infant weight check about every three days until the mother's milk supply is stable and the infant is gaining well.

A summary of interventions for flat or inverted nipples appears in **Table 2-1**. Clinicians may select one or more interventions that have the highest potential to remedy the particular situation.

Table 2-1. Summary of Flat/Inverted Nipple Interventions

Intervention	Pros	Cons
Pre-Birth		
Prenatal correction	Familiarizes mothers with handling her breasts	Is generally ineffective
Prenatal suction correction with Niplette	Is an effective tissue expander	Has the potential for pain and bleeding if too much suction is applied
Prenatal surgical correction	Is very effective in correcting inverted nipples	Has a high potential for severing ducts within the nipple and impeding breastfeeding
Post-Birth		
Cold compress prior to feeding	Will cause contraction of erector muscles	May not be sufficient to affect an inverted nipple or provide enough graspable tissue for some infants
Pull and roll nipple prior to feeding	Is a fast and easy method to evert a nipple	May not stay everted long enough for some infants or provide sufficient graspable tissue
Pop out nipple prior to feeding	Is a fast and easy method to evert a nipple	May not be effective with inverted nipples or nipples tightly tethered to underlying tissue
Breast pump	Extends nipple away from areola, stretching it into nipple tunnel	Distributes vacuum over a large area; causes nipple swelling; does not provide steady or controllable vacuum
10mL syringe	Is easy, inexpensive, effective method to evert nipple	May not be allowed by some hospitals that restrict the use of non-FDA approved devices
Evert-it Nipple Enhancer	Is an FDA approved device for everting flat nipples	Have little data as to its effectiveness
Latch Assist	Is an FDA approved device for everting flat nipples	Have little data as to its effectiveness
Breast shells	May help reduce areolar edema surrounding nipple	May cause tissue damage if areolar edema is present and shells are worn for extended periods of time,
Reverse pressure softening	Helps reveal nipple enveloped by edematous areola	May not expose enough of the nipple for infant to grasp
Teacup hold	May provide sufficient tissue for a good latch	Is not effective on an engorged breast or edematous areola
Dimple ring	Is a simple device to hold open a dimpled nipple for air drying	May be difficult to locate
Nipple shield	Is useful if no other techniques or devices are effective in facilitating a good latch	May be difficult for some infants to learn to latch without the shield

A sample plan for breastfeeding with flat or inverted nipples is shown in **Box 2-2.**

Box 2-2. Sample Breastfeeding Plan for Flat and Inverted Nipples

Prior to latch	Try cold compresses, nipple rolling, and/or popping out the nipple followed by the teacup hold.
If the infant still cannot latch	Try modified syringe to evert nipple prior to each feeding; use modified syringe several times between feedings to continue stretching the nipple; can try breast shells between feedings.
If the areola is edematous	Use reverse pressure softening technique prior to each feeding.
If the infant still cannot latch	Try nipple shields for each feeding; apply the shield, have mother hand express colostrum or milk into teat. If she cannot do this, prefill the teat with colostrum or milk using a periodontal syringe.

SORE NIPPLES

Sore nipples are a common problem reported by new mothers. Pain or fear of pain is a frequent reason that many mothers avoid breastfeeding or abandon it early (Cricco-Lizza, 2004; Hurley, Black, Papas, & Quigg, 2008; Wambach & Koehn, 2004). Sore nipples typically reside in the top two or three reasons that mothers terminate breastfeeding (Murimi, Dodge, Pope, & Erickson, 2010). This is especially true in the low income as well as the African American population of mothers (Alexander, Dowling, & Furman, 2010). Identified as a major impediment to breastfeeding, sore nipples, while a common problem, ranks high on the list of problems to avoid or remediate quickly. The incidence of sore nipples varies widely. Data reported in the literature on the incidence of sore nipples range from none at six days post delivery (Humenick & van Steenkiste, 1983) to 96% of breastfeeding mothers experiencing nipple discomfort at some time during the first six weeks postpartum (Ziemer et al., 1990). The concept of soreness or pain is subjective, and studies on nipple pain vary in their methodology, leading to a wide incidence range. Clinically, most mothers report some kind of sensation when they first put their infant to breast, even if it is nothing more than a fleeting discomfort at latch.

There are many aspects of nipple pain, such as transient pain at latch, sustained pain during a feeding, persistent nipple pain over a prolonged period of time, pain between feedings, and burning pain. Degrees of pain range from mild sensitivity to excruciating. Sore nipples are a frequently reported reason for early termination of breastfeeding (Ahluwalia, Morrow, & Hsia, 2005; Neifert & Seacat, 1986; West, 1980; Yeung, Pennell, Leung, & Hall, 1981). Nipple pain (of any definition) has been reported to occur from the 2nd to the 15th postpartum day, continuing in some mothers through 90 days (Drewett, Kahn, Parkhurst, & Whiteley, 1987). It peaks in intensity from day two or three (Hewat & Ellis, 1987; Newton, 1952) up to days 4 through 7 (Ziemer et al., 1990).

In a study of the nipple pain experiences of 69 women, Heads and Higgins (1995) reported that about 75% of the mothers had pain at the outset of breastfeeding, which declined sharply to 22% following letdown and the establishment of breastfeeding. Hill and Humenick (1993) described the daily occurrence of pain during latch for the first 14 days in 155 first- and second-time breastfeeding mothers, as well as the occurrence of pain severe enough to disrupt breastfeeding over the course of the first six weeks. Virtually all of the mothers experienced some level of discomfort when the baby first latched on (as also noted by L'Esperance, 1980). The maximum level of latch-on pain was reached by day five in 73.8% of the mothers. Latch-on pain and breast engorgement have been positively correlated, showing that mothers experiencing more engorgement experienced more latch-on pain (Briggs, 2003).

The incidence of mothers experiencing nipple pain severe enough to interfere with breastfeeding ranged from 42.3% at week one to 12.4% at week six. Mothers experiencing nipple pain severe enough to interfere with their desire to continue breastfeeding was significantly associated with latch-on pain at weeks one and two. Up to one-third of mothers experiencing nipple pain and trauma may change to alternate feeding methods within the first six weeks postpartum. Coca, Gamba, de Souza e Silva, and Abrao (2009) conducted a case control study in 146 recently delivered mothers, showing that factors associated with nipple trauma included engorged breasts and nipples that were flat or malformed.

Unfortunately, according to two recent studies, nipple pain can persist past the first few days. The first sample was from Minneapolis, Minnesota. In this sample, 50% of women had nipple pain at five weeks (McGovern et al., 2006). Another study from Toronto, Canada, had similar results. In this study, 52% of mothers reported cracked or sore nipples at two months postpartum (Ansara et al., 2005).

Mothers with nipple anomalies had a significantly higher incidence of nipple trauma than mothers with normal nipples. Mothers who experience nipple pain also suffer from high levels of psychological distress (Amir et al., 1997), confirming that clinical support to improve nipple pain is important during the early days and weeks postpartum if breastfeeding is to continue. Pain or the anticipation of pain can delay or disrupt the milk-ejection reflex, which can set in motion a cascade of undesirable side effects, leading to ineffective milk transfer, residual milk build-up, more or extended engorgement, and coming full circle to more nipple pain (Newton & Newton, 1948).

Ziemer and Pigeon (1993) described nipple skin changes in 20 breastfeeding mothers during the first week of lactation. They speculated that not all nipple pain and damage is caused from faulty positioning or sucking and that some of the changes and discomfort mentioned by mothers may be part of the normal process of initiating breastfeeding. The authors probably put forth this assumption because all of the mothers in their study demonstrated some type of change in the nipple during the study period. Changes and damage to the nipple skin were almost always confined to the face or tip of the nipple, suggesting that normal changes as well as actual damage was due to suction, not friction from the action of the tongue. One mother experienced damage at the base of the nipple where it attaches to the areola. The skin appeared split, suggesting that the limits of elasticity in this particular nipple may have been reached. Ninety percent of the women experienced pain. Pain intensity did not differ significantly among women with fair or darker skin. Magnified photographs of the nipple tip in all women studied showed visible skin changes during the study period. The tip of the nipple prior to the start of breastfeeding was light pink and typically showed a papillar (small bumps) appearance, with small lines and crevices uniquely distributed over the surface. Ten different changes were observed over time:

- **Erythema** (reddening or inflamed areas): This peaked on day three.
- **Edema** (swelling) of the nipple and papillar bumps: Occurred in all of the women and peaked on day five.
- **Fissures:** For 65% of the mothers, some of the fissures widened and became raw, peaking on day five.
- **Blisters:** 80% of the mothers had small blisters that could have been papillae filled with fluid; occurred on day three.

Also seen were eschar (scabs), white patches, peeling, dark patches, pus, and ecchymosis (bruising or bleeding under the skin).

On day five, an average of 25% of the erectile portion of the nipple skin was involved. Little-to-no damage was seen on the areola. The presence of inflamed areas and scabbing were associated with increased intensity of pain.

Positioning or proper nipple/areolar placement in the infant's mouth was not evaluated in this study; however, nipple skin changes were seen to occur right from the start of breastfeeding. When the epidermis is injured, there is an initial reaction of inflammation, with redness, swelling, and pain. This may be what many mothers describe as sore nipples. If, however, the damage is severe, a process is set in motion where fluid and cells escape from dilated blood vessels, and exudate (oozing of fluid) occurs and dries, forming a scab if there is nothing covering the damaged skin. These normal changes may be responsible for the common complaints of mothers describing some amount of nipple sensitivity or discomfort, while severe nipple pain may represent an exaggeration or extension of these changes.

Positioning: Proper Nipple/Areolar Placement

Gunther (1945) was one of the earliest authors to associate severe nipple pain and damage with the position of the baby at the breast. She described two common types of damage as erosive (petechial) and ulcerative (fissure). Woolridge (1986b) described frictional trauma and suction lesions as the two main physical sources of nipple pain (as opposed to dermatologic or infective causes). Frictional trauma is thought to be caused by inadequate amounts of breast tissue being drawn into the baby's mouth, resulting in poor milk transfer and distortion of the nipple. Rather than being compressed and extending to twice its resting length, the nipple/areolar complex is not formed into a teat, and the nipple skin can become abraded or actually pinched into a compression stripe. A nipple that is creased in a horizontal, vertical, or oblique manner has the potential for both significant pain and skin breakdown (caused by both compression and suction concentrated on the distorted area).

Trauma from suction has been related to the application of continuous suction that is not relieved by periodic swallowing. Righard (1996) provided further insight into the effect of faulty sucking on nipple pain. Of the 52 mother/baby pairs referred for breastfeeding problems, 94% had a pattern of superficial nipple sucking, where the infant sucked only on the nipple tip, failing to draw the nipple/areola complex deep into the mouth. Of the 94% of mother/baby pairs with the superficial sucking pattern, 33% of the mothers complained of sore nipples. An interesting finding in this study was that infants using pacifiers more often had a superficial sucking pattern at the breast than nonusers of pacifiers.

Nipple pain from faulty mechanics of infant sucking, either poor latch or failure to form a teat (Righard, 1998; Widstrom & Thingstrom-Paulsson, 1993), can occur quickly, with mothers experiencing nipple pain and damage prior to discharge from the hospital. Blair, Cadwell, Turner-Maffei, and Brimdyr (2003) studied 95 mothers reporting nipple pain within 10 days of giving birth. They looked at a number of latching and positioning behaviors, such as rooting, gape, seal, and suck, the infant's head position, flanging of the lips, infant body position, the infant's height relative to the breast, infant's body rotation, and the infant's cheek line. Their results showed that nipple pain was related to positioning and latching errors, but that no single isolated part of the positioning and latch sequence was more related to pain than another. Clinicians, therefore, need to assess all elements of the positioning, latching, and sucking processes. Mothers in this study experienced slightly less pain if their infant latched properly, with a wide open mouth and the lips sealed appropriately on the breast. The latching process in this study seemed to have a relationship to the mother's stated level of pain. Six specific types of nipple trauma were distributed among the mothers in this study: (1) 64.4% presented with fissures, (2) 53.3% with erythema, (3) 51.1% with crusting/scabs, (4) 32.2% with swelling, (5) 4.4% with blisters or blebs, and (6) 1.1% with exudate.

It is interesting to note that Ziemer and Pigeon (1993) also reported a 65% rate of fissures in their description of causes of nipple pain. It could be speculated that faulty positioning, latching, and sucking mechanics could place enough stress on the normal anatomic features of the nipple (papillae and fissures on the face of the nipple) to cause erosion or a break in the skin integrity. The disruption of the skin surface by suction or friction, concomitant stretching or rupturing of the skin within the fissures, and destruction of the underlying skin layers may move the mother on a continuum from minor discomfort to macerated and bleeding nipple wounds if interventions do not rectify the problem.

Improper nipple position within the infant's mouth has long been thought to contribute to sore and damaged nipples. Jacobs et al. (2007) used ultrasound to measure the distance between the tip of the nipple and the junction of the hard and soft palates after study infants painlessly drew the nipple/areola into their mouths. Only 25% of correctly latched infants drew in the nipple as far as the hard/soft palate junction. The median distance between the tip of the nipple and this junction was 5 mm, and the nipple showed a range of movement during breastfeeding of 4.0 ± 1.3 mm. Nipple position did not have a significant impact on milk transfer in the study infants. Excessive nipple movement and positioning outside these ranges may be associated with sucking problems and be predictive of nipple pain. An incidental observation of the slow-motion video tapes taken during this study confirmed the Geddes et al. (2008a) observations that the tongue in its most upward position held the nipple in contact with the palate, but did not mechanically squeeze out any milk into the mouth. When the tongue moved downward, milk was seen exiting the nipple.

Ankyloglossia

Ankyloglossia (tongue-tie) can restrict or alter the movement of the tongue. This has the potential to inhibit the nipple/areola from being drawn far enough into the mouth to prevent pain and promote optimal milk transfer. Nipple pain is a common complaint of mothers whose infants are diagnosed with ankyloglossia (Hogan, Westcott, & Griffiths, 2005; Ballard, Auer, & Khoury, 2002; Messner, Lalakea, Aby, MacMahon, & Blair, 2000; Srinivasan, Dobrich, Mitnick, & Feldman, 2006; Wallace & Clark, 2006). Ballard and colleagues (2002) assessed nipple pain on an analog scale of 1 to 10, with 10 representing severe or intolerable pain, in mothers whose infants were identified as having ankyloglossia. Significant ankyloglossia was diagnosed on the first or second day of life in 3.2% of the entire inpatient breastfeeding population seen during the study period. All of these inpatient mother/infant pairs exhibited either poor latch or maternal nipple pain while still in the hospital. Mean nipple pain scores were 6.9 ± 2.31 before the frenuloplasty and 1.2 ± 1.52 after frenuloplasty. When ankyloglossia was diagnosed on outpatient mother/infant pairs, more severe complications were present that included damaged and infected nipples. The combination of poor latch and maternal nipple pain are frequent presenting complaints in situations where ankyloglossia is ultimately diagnosed.

Griffiths (2004) and Wallace and Clark (2006) also noticed that in addition to poor latch and nipple pain, continuous feeding was another common presenting factor. Seventy-seven percent of the mothers in this study of 215 infants with ankyloglossia experienced nipple pain and trauma that included nipple bleeding. Once division of the frenulum occurred, most mothers reported improved feeding and a reduction in nipple pain. Nipple pain was so severe in some of these mothers that they used a nipple shield until tongue division could take place. Srinivasan and colleagues (2006) measured changes in latch and maternal nipple pain following frenotomy (clipping the frenulum) in 27 infants. Mothers' nipple pain was assessed by the Short-Form McGill Pain Questionnaire that has two subsets, the Pain Rating Index that rates the intensity of various types of pain and the Present Pain Index, which asks the mother to rate her overall pain on a scale of 0 (lowest) to 5 (highest). Frenotomy decreased nipple pain almost immediately. Optimal latches postfrenotomy resulted in a larger decrease in nipple pain than when postfrenotomy latches were still suboptimal. This study showed that improvement in nipple pain was associated with the quality of latch achieved after frenotomy. When frenotomy does not significantly improve latch, nipple pain or discomfort may persist. This may happen if an insufficient amount of the frenulum was released or with a Type 3 or Type 4 tongue tie that are more difficult to visualize and treat.

Geddes et al. (2008b) reported that release of the frenulum altered tongue movement as imaged by ultrasound during breastfeeding. Infants with ankyloglossia showed two types of sucking dynamics, one type pinched the nipple tip, placing it a large distance from the junction of the hard and soft palate. The other type of sucking pinched the nipple at its base, placing the nipple tip in close proximity to the hard/soft palate junction. Frenotomy reduced the extent of nipple distortion and significantly relieved nipple pain experienced by mothers. Dollberg, Botzer, Grunis, and Mimouni (2006) recruited 25 mothers with sore nipples whose infants were diagnosed with ankyloglossia. Using standardized latch and pain scores, a significant decrease in nipple pain was seen immediately after frenotomy. Sham frenotomies in this study did not result in improved nipple pain.

In a study by Khoo, Dabbas, Sudhakaran, Ade-Ajayi, and Patel (2009), 62 infants with ankyloglossia underwent frenulotomy (surgical release of the lingual frenulum; also called frenectomy, frenulectomy, and frenuloplasty). Eighty-four percent of mothers presented with nipple pain and 52% with nipple trauma. Three months after the procedure 78% of the mothers were still breastfeeding, feed lengths had significantly decreased, and time between feeds had significantly increased. Those mothers with the highest amount of nipple pain pre-frenulotomy showed the highest likelihood of continued breastfeeding at three months. Correcting ankyloglossia had a striking affect not only on comfort levels, but was associated with the avoidance of the abandonment of breastfeeding due to unremitting pain at feedings.

Not all clinicians agree on the treatment of ankyloglossia. Messner and colleagues (2000) surveyed four disciplines–otolaryngologists, pediatricians, lactation consultants, and speech pathologists–to determine their opinions of the relationship between ankyloglossia and feeding, speech, and social/mechanical problems. Results showed large differences of opinion among the various disciplines, with pediatricians being the least likely to recommend surgery. If surgery is not to be performed or if there is a delay in finding a clinician to perform a frenotomy, then a feeding plan will need to be devised to assure adequate intake and preserve the mother's milk supply (**Box 2-3**).

Box 2-3. Feeding Plan Considerations Prior to Frenotomy (or if Frenotomy Will Not be Done)

When positioning the infant, use positions that encourage forward and downward movement of the infant's tongue, such as placing the infant ventrally (semi-prone), completely vertical, or in an upright clutch hold.
Modifications surrounding latch-on can include: stroking the infant's tongue down and forward with an index finger prior to latch, providing chin or jaw support to help maintain the latch, using techniques to evert nipples if they are flat, and shaping the breast for a deep latch.
A nipple shield can be used if the nipples are too sore or damaged for comfortable feeding.
Mothers may need to pump their breasts following each feeding to assure an adequate milk supply and to provide a supplement if the infant is unable to transfer sufficient amounts of milk while feeding at the breast.
Infant weight should be check every three days until an adequate pattern of weight gain is established. Even if a tongue-tied infant can feed at the breast, he may not feed at optimum efficiency and may require pumped milk supplements.
Close attention should be paid to articulation achievements as the infant/child begins to vocalize.

Other Causes of Nipple Pain

While much of the nipple pain experienced by mothers may be relieved by correcting positioning and attachment at the breast, assessment and correction of technique does not relieve all nipple pain (Cadwell, Turner-Maffei, Blair, Brimdyr, & McInerney, 2004; Henderson, Stamp, & Pincombe, 2001). Cadwell et al. (2004) conducted a study that assessed and corrected positioning and attachment in mothers experiencing nipple pain. Ten percent of the mothers recruited showed no improvement in nipple condition in spite of clinical interventions known to improve sore nipples.

McClellan et al. (2008) demonstrated that despite help with positioning and attachment, the infants of mothers with persistent nipple pain applied significantly stronger vacuums and transferred less milk than infants not causing pain. Their data revealed that infants causing pain exerted vacuums that were more than 50% stronger during active sucking and more than double during pausing when compared to infants not causing pain. In these infants, all components of the suck cycle were stronger, with the baseline seal at the breast 61% stronger and the peak vacuum 31% stronger than infants who were not causing nipple pain. Interventions to reduce these strong vacuums are unknown, but techniques, such as more frequent feeding to reduce strong sucking due to hunger, changes in positioning, such as to ventral positioning, sucking on the mother's finger prior to each feeding, and/or use of a nipple shield, can be tried to help alleviate some of the pain.

Treatments for Sore Nipples

Remedies for sore nipples have been written about since the 17th century when plasters, poultices, and ointments were applied topically to provide comfort for the mother. A plethora of nipple soreness treatments abound from simple warm water soaks to multi-ingredient commercial preparations (**Box 2-4**), with no single agent being clearly superior to others (Morland-Schultz & Hill, 2005).

Box 2-4. Nipple Soreness Treatments

Warm wet compress	Saline soaks	Expressed breastmilk
Wet teabags	Lanolin	Olive oil
Chlorhexidine (0.2%) spray	Vitamin E oil	Hydrogel dressings
Peppermint water	Peppermint gel	A & D ointment
Triple antibiotic	Herbal preparations	Lotrimin AF
All purpose nipple ointment	Neosporin	Bacitracin
Homeopathic remedies	Micatin	Monistat
Commercial nipple creams	Laser therapy	

A number of systematic reviews and a few randomized clinical trials of sore nipple interventions have yielded inconclusive results. Several studies with small numbers of mothers have compared various treatments, with some yielding better results than others. **Table 2-2** uses selected studies to compare various topical agents for the treatment or prevention of nipple pain.

Table 2-2. Comparison of Topical Agents for Treatment or Prevention of Nipple Pain

Agent	Positive results	Equivalent results	Negative results
Expressed mother's milk (EMM)	Superior to lanolin (Mohammadzadeh, Farhat, & Esmaeily, 2005)	Equivalent to lanolin (Hewit & Ellis, 1987)	Inferior to warm water compresses (Buchko et al, 1994; Pugh et al., 1996) Inferior to keeping nipples dry and clean (Akkuzu & Taskin, 2000) Inferior to lanolin (Coca & Abrao, 2008) Inferior to peppermint water (Manizheh et al., 2007a)
Tea bag compress		Equivalent to lanolin in neither preventing nor reducing soreness (Riordan, 1985) Equivalent to warm water compress (Lavergne, 1997)	Inferior to warm water compresses (Buchko et al., 1994)
Warm water compress	Superior to tea bags or EMM (Buchko et al., 1994) Superior to lanolin and EMM (Pugh et al., 1996)	Equivalent to tea bags (Lavergne, 1997)	Inferior to keeping nipples dry and clean (Akkuzu & Taskin, 2000)

Lanolin	Superior to no treatment after five days (Spangler & Hildebrandt, 1993) Superior to EMM (Coca & Abrao, 2008)	Equivalent to EMM (Hewat & Ellis, 1987) Equivalent to tea bags in neither preventing nor reducing soreness (Riordan, 1985)	Inferior to warm water compresses (Pugh et al., 1996) Inferior to hydrogel dressings (Dodd & Chalmers, 2003) Inferior to EMM (Mohammadzadeh et al., 2005) Inferior to peppermint gel (Manizheh et al, 2007b)
Hydrogel dressing	Superior to lanolin (Dodd & Chalmers, 2003)		
Peppermint gel	Superior to lanolin (Manizheh et al., 2007b)		
Peppermint water	Superior to EMM (Manizheh et al, 2007a)		

Adapted from (Lochner et al., 2009).

Warm water compresses may offer mothers relief from soreness, as warmth promotes comfort and may also promote healing by enhancing blood flow to the wound and facilitating the removal of waste products. Some clinicians recommend adding ¼-½ teaspoon salt per quart of warm water and soaking the breast/nipple area in a small amount of the salt water for 10 minutes or so, and then patting dry.

Plant Extracts

Plant extracts have been widely used as topical applications for wound-healing. Many of the plants used to improve skin conditions or heal wounds share a common characteristic: they produce flavonoid compounds with phenolic components. These phytochemicals are highly reactive and serve to neutralize free radicals or initiate biological effects.

Green Tea. Green tea contains a group of polyphenol compounds called catechins that can facilitate natural wound healing (Hsu, 2005). Keratinocytes are epidermal cells which synthesize keratin and undergo characteristic changes as they move upward from the basal layers of the epidermis to the cornified (horny) layer of the skin. They undergo programmed cell death to form the cornified layer, which serves as a barrier to mechanical injury, microbial invasion, and water loss. At certain concentrations, green tea polyphenols have been shown to stimulate aged keratinocytes, energizing cell division and DNA synthesis, and potentially reducing the healing time of epidermal wounds (Hsu et al., 2003). This may be why some mothers enjoy relief of their nipple wounds from the use of certain types of tea bags.

Peppermint. Peppermint (*Mentha piperita*) exhibits a calming and numbing effect, especially when used to relieve skin irritations (Blumenthal, Goldberg, & Brinckmann, 2000). Peppermint increases tissue flexibility, improving its resistance to cracking (Schelz, Molnar, & Hohmann, 2006). Peppermint oil demonstrates strong antibacterial activity and is anti-inflammatory. As an antioxidant, it is a potent free-radical scavenger, and it possesses both fungistatic and fungicidal qualities (Mimica-Dukić, Bozin, Soković, Mihajlović, & Matavuli, 2003; Mimica-Dukic & Bozin, 2008).

Manizheh and colleagues (2007b) conducted a randomized, double-blind study in Iran on 163 mothers divided into three groups: those using purified lanolin, those using a peppermint gel, and a third group using a placebo gel. Mothers were instructed to rub the preparation on their nipples following each breastfeeding to potentially prevent sore or damaged nipples. The peppermint gel was composed of carbopol 934, 0.2% propyl paraben, 0.1% methyl paraben, 15 ml glycerin (as a humectant to retain moisture), and 0.2 ml peppermint oil. The rate of nipple cracks was 22.6% in the placebo group, 6.9% in the lanolin group, and 3.8% in the peppermint group. At week six, 27% of the placebo group reported use of infant formula in addition to breastmilk, 13% of the lanolin group used formula, and 5.6% of the peppermint group added formula to their infant's diet.

The use of peppermint gel prophylactically was more effective than the use of peppermint water on the nipples. But Manizheh et al. (2007a) found that even peppermint water used on nipples was three times more effective in preventing nipple cracks than expressed breastmilk on the nipples (27% expressed breastmilk vs. 9% peppermint water). The peppermint-gel preparation was probably more effective than the peppermint water because its gel base promoted longer contact with the nipple epidermis, allowing prolonged action of the peppermint properties, and it retained moisture better. Peppermint in both studies was used prophylactically in the prevention of nipple wounds, not on existing nipple injuries, although the healing properties of peppermint would be expected to expedite wound healing. Peppermint gel was also effective in reducing nipple pain.

Olive oil. While olive oil as a topical agent for sore nipples is anecdotally used, data on olive oil for this application is lacking. Robinson (2002) anecdotally discusses the use of olive oil on sore nipples, noting that the product in her practice is effective, inexpensive, easily accessible, and useful in promoting the healing of sore nipples. Olive oil has been used extensively in skin care and skin diseases.

Preparations of olive oil have historically been used externally for wound dressing and for minor burns and psoriasis. Olive oil and compounds containing olive oil have demonstrated some efficacy for the treatment of several skin conditions, including eczematous dermatoses, rosacea, and wound healing (Ahurjai & Natsheh, 2003; Baumann, 2007; Saary et al., 2005). The oil has numerous biologically active components, including fatty acids, tocopherols, and carotenoids. Skin-related attributes associated with olive oil include antioxidant and anti-inflammatory activity, as well as protection against ultraviolet (UV) radiation.

Hydrophilic phenols are the most abundant natural antioxidants of virgin olive oil, and important biological properties (antioxidant, anti-inflammatory, chemopreventive, and anti-cancer) have been attributed to these phenols (Servili et al., 2009). The composition of olive oil includes tocopherols (an excellent source of Vitamin E) and the unsaturated fatty acids - oleic, linoleic, and linolenic acid.

Olive oil is a natural source for significant quantities of squalene, which is the main component of skin surface polyunsaturated lipids. The topical application of squalene is advantageous for the skin as an emollient and antioxidant and for hydration and antitumor activities (Huang, Lin, & Fang, 2009). As an emollient, squalene is quickly and efficiently absorbed deep into the skin, restoring suppleness and flexibility.

Olive oil has the ability, however, to block pores, and a small risk of infection exists from the application of contaminated olive oil to the skin. Al-Waili (2005) examined a honey, beeswax, and olive oil mixture in terms of the growth of *Staphylococcus aureus* and *Candida albicans* on growth media. This particular mixture of ingredients is useful in the treatment of diaper dermatitis, psoriasis, and eczema. Results of the study showed that no growth of *S. aureus* or *C. albicans* grew on media containing only honey, whereas mild to moderate growth was obtained on media containing only olive oil or only beeswax. However, media with the mixture showed a clear zone of growth inhibition.

Ozonated olive oil has been shown to be effective in animal models for accelerating wound repair and in promoting granulation tissue formation, a step in the healing process (Kim et al., 2009; Sakazaki et al., 2007). Olive oil is treated with gaseous ozone to produce a treatment with advantages over traditional anti-microbial agents. Microbes have a poor defense mechanism against strong oxidants. This is why there is no bacterial resistance to ozone, unlike other antibacterial agents. These oils have a greater advantage over commonly used antiseptics and ointments due to their wide range of activities during all phases of the healing process. Ozonated olive oil is available in commercial preparations, but no studies could be found on its use in nipple wound healing.

MEBO. Moist exposed burn ointment (MEBO) is a Chinese herbal formulation that has been used for the management of partial-thickness burns in China for many years. It contains b-sitosterol, baicalin (an anti-inflammatory and anti-fungal), berberine (an anti-bacterial and anti-fungal), in a base of beeswax and sesame oil. Li et al. (2000) report the successful treatment of 260 cases of nipple fissures, with healing in 3-12 days.

Dry Wound Healing

Dry wound healing (air drying, sunlight, sun lamp, hair dryer, heat from a light bulb) has been historically advocated for many years. It was thought that continued tissue destruction and slower wound healing would occur if the nipples remained wet and that rapid drying would prevent this. However, this assumption has not proven to be correct, as moist wound healing is more effective.

Treatment of nipple fissures or damage is consistent with treating other types of skin fissures, which is to increase the moisture content of the skin and reduce further drying by applying an emollient to the damaged area (Sharp, 1992). An emollient is soothing and provides a moisture barrier that slows the evaporation of moisture naturally present in the skin, eliminating further drying and cracking. Scab formation does not occur when using moist-wound healing.

Rapid drying causes the stratum corneum to shrink in an irregular manner, placing tension on a layer of fragile tissue. The use of an emollient, such as USP-modified anhydrous lanolin, allows the contours of the stratum corneum to return to normal, enhancing the movement of cells across the wound as it heals. Sharp (1992) delineates a difference between surface-skin moisture and internal moisture, stating that although a mother may pat the nipple area with a clean cloth to remove surface wetness, rapid drying can deplete the skin of internal moisture. He compares this to the act of licking dry chapped lips, which sets up a rapid wet-to-dry process that worsens the original condition.

Commercial Nipple Creams

While most commercial nipple cream preparations cause no harm, not all contain active and inactive ingredients that are safe for use with infants. The Environmental Working Group's cosmetic safety database[1], Skin Deep, lists 31 commercial nipple creams for breastfeeding mothers. This data base rates each preparation as 0-2 low hazard, 3-6 moderate hazard, and 7-10 high hazard based on an analysis of each ingredient for carcinogenic potential, developmental/reproductive toxicity, violations, restrictions, warnings, neurotoxicity, endocrine disruptions, allergies/immunotoxicity, organ toxicity, and multiple/additive exposure sources. Twelve products scored 0, 11 products scored 1, 3 products scored 2, 1 product scored 4, 1 product scored 5, and 3 products scored 6. It is important for clinicians to be aware of these products and to find out which, if any, mothers are using. Checking this database will alert clinicians and mothers to products that are suitable or unsuitable for use relative to ingredient safety.

On May 23, 2008, the FDA issued a warning[2] that a particular commercial nipple cream should not be used because it contained chlorphenesin, a skeletal muscle relaxant that depresses the central nervous system and causes respiratory depression. It also contained phenoxyethanol, a preservative that can cause central nervous system depression, as well as

1 http://www.cosmeticsdatabase.com/browse.php?category=nipplecream

2 http://www.fda.gov/NewsEvents/Newsroom/PressAnnouncements/2008/ucm116900.htm

vomiting and diarrhea. Chlorphenesin has the potential to harm the mother by causing dermatitis, which can exacerbate the drying and cracking of the nipple skin.

Box 2-5 provides sample intervention plans for sore nipples.

Box 2-5. Sample Intervention Plans for Sore Nipples

Preventive strategies
• Use optimal positioning. Assess latch, suck, and swallowing and correct positioning if necessary.
• Use a modified syringe, nipple rolling, or tea cup hold to assist with latch if nipples are flat.
• Place infant in ventral position (prone) for gravity assistance, optimal ventilation, and advantageous use of primitive neonatal reflexes (Colson, Meek, & Hawdon, 2008).
• Check to make sure the infant's mouth is open to 160°, with lips flared outwards and neck slightly extended.
• If pumping, assure the flange is large enough to prevent nipple strangulation in flange tunnel.
• Provide relief from engorgement.
• Avoid pacifiers until breastfeeding is well established.
• Correct ankyloglossia if present.
• Apply peppermint water or peppermint gel to nipples after each early feeding.
When nipples are already sore
In addition to the above measures, the following preparations may be tried for soothing, pain relief, and healing:
• Warm water compresses
• Warm green tea bag compresses
• Peppermint water or gel
• Olive oil
• Commercial nipple creams with a 0-2 rating on the Environmental Working Group's cosmetic safety database
• Nipple shield if nothing else is working and the mother verbalizes her desire to stop breastfeeding

When More Extensive Interventions May Be Necessary

Cracked Nipples/Bacterial Infection

Discomfort and pain due to physical forces on the nipple can often be remedied through correcting and optimizing the mechanics of breastfeeding (Renfrew, Woolridge, & McGill, 2000). However, if mothers have nipple anomalies, have an infant with uncorrected ankyloglossia, or experience faulty infant positioning or sucking at breast for a period of time, nipple pain may persist or worsen. If a break in the skin surface occurs, other factors may become involved and more extensive interventions may be necessary. Once the integrity of the skin has been disrupted, there is a tendency for colonization by bacterial and fungal species.

Nipple wounds are easily and frequently contaminated by *S. aureus*, a common bacterial resident of the skin. Livingstone, Willis, and Berkowitz (1996) showed that mothers with infants younger than one month who presented with severe nipple pain and damage (cracks, fissures, ulcers, or exudates) had a 64% chance of having a positive bacterial skin culture and a 54% chance of having *S. aureus* impetigo vulgaris colonization. Impetigo vulgaris is a bacterial skin infection caused by staphylococci or streptococci, with yellow to red weeping and crusted or pustular lesions. The term vulgaris refers to the common form of this infection. Among mothers with sore nipples, if there was a break in the nipple integument (skin) associated with cracks, fissures, ulcers, or pus, the chance of having *S. aureus* colonization was 36%. This was five times higher than in mothers without a break in the integument.

Repetitive trauma to the nipple skin is thought to overcome the natural barriers to infection, and once bacterial contamination has occurred, a delay in wound healing may follow. Livingstone and Stringer (1999) studied 84 mothers with sore, cracked nipples and positive *S. aureus* cultures. Four different treatments were compared in a randomized clinical trial: review of basic breastfeeding techniques alone, topical treatment with 2% mupirocin ointment applied to the nipples after each breastfeed, topical fusidic acid ointment applied to the nipples post-feed, or oral cloxacillin/erythromycin 500 mg every six hours for 10 days. Following five to seven days of treatment, only 8% of mothers showed improvement in the optimal breastfeeding technique group, 16% improved with topical mupirocin, 29% improved with topical fusidic acid, and 79% improved with oral antibiotics. The risk of developing mastitis was 25% among mothers who were not treated systemically compared to 5% for mothers who received oral antibiotics. Once the nipple skin barrier is breeched, a progression of pathologic sequelae can occur, leading to the need for more aggressive interventions (**Box 2-6**).

Box 2-6. Progression of Possible Pathologic Sequelae in Cracked Nipples

•	Nipple skin becomes a reservoir of *S. aureus*.
•	Nipple trauma breeches nipple skin integrity.
•	*S. aureus* strains penetrate superficial layers of broken epidermis.
•	Toxins produced cause inflammation, epidermal separation, and blisters.
•	Blisters open causing erosions that become covered by a yellow, crusted exudate.
•	Pain occurs sufficient to inhibit let-down or reduce milk transfer leading to milk stasis.
•	Infection occurs in the ascending lactiferous duct.
•	Mastitis develops if infection is not treated.
•	Abscess may develop if mastitis is not treated.

Biofilm Formation

Due to the link between severe nipple soreness and colonization and infection of the nipple by *S. aureus*, careful washing of the nipple with soap and water and the application of mupirocin 2% ointment (Bactroban) may be effective in the early stages of the infection (Livingstone et al., 1996). Bacteria have the ability to grow in colonies and protect the colony with a coating called a biofilm (**Figure 2-1**). Biofilms may potentially be stimulated by saliva when a baby feeds at the breast (Stewart & Costerton, 2001). In order to disrupt this protective biofilm, washing the nipple wound with soap and water once a day, followed by a coating of mupirocin may penetrate the biofilm, promote wound healing, and prevent progression to an infection (Ryan, 2007).

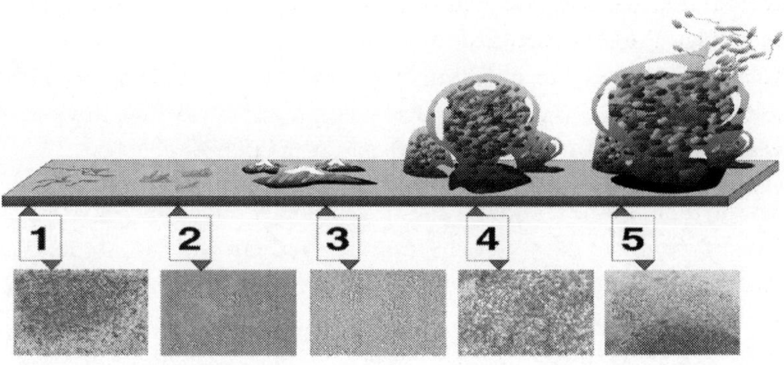

Figure 2-1. Biofilm Formation
Five stages of biofilm development. Stage 1: initial attachment; Stage 2: irreversible attachment; Stage 3: maturation I; Stage 4: maturation II; Stage 5: dispersion. Each stage of development in the diagram is paired with a photomicrograph of a developing P. aeruginosa biofilm. All photomicrographs are shown to same scale. *From (Monroe, 2007). Reprinted from Public Library of Science journal, an open access publication.*

Biofilms also develop on pacifiers and can serve as a reservoir for infection and re-infection of damaged nipples. Comina et al. (2006) studied 25 pacifiers used in daycare centers (9 silicone and 16 latex). Biofilm presence was seen on 80% of the pacifiers, with latex pacifiers being more contaminated than silicone ones. The two primary genera that were isolated included *Staphylococcus* and *Candida.* Pacifiers should be avoided if at all possible in the early weeks of breastfeeding, especially if there is a break in the nipple skin. If used, pacifiers should be washed frequently and thoroughly, including the plastic part that covers the mouth.

Use of Topical Steroids, Systemic Antibiotics, and Topical Anti-Fungals

Because much nipple pain may stem from inflammation, topical application of low- to medium-strength steroids may provide welcome relief. No adverse effects have been reported when these types of preparations are used sparingly as thin coats to the nipples (Huggins & Billion, 1993). Systemic antibiotics may need to be added to the treatment regime if exudate is seen, erythema increases, or dry-scab formation is absent. Persistent sore nipples may be a combination of yeast and bacterial infection, causing difficulty in differentiating the offending organism.

Some clinicians will use miconazole 2% as the antifungal preparation, in combination with mupirocin and a topical steroid to ensure the best results (Porter & Schach, 2004). Interventions should assure that repetitive trauma to the nipple is corrected. With persistent or recurrent infections, it may be necessary to treat the infant with nasal mupirocin because the infant may function as a *S. aureus* carrier and a vector for infecting or re-infecting the mother (Amir, Garland, & Lumley, 2006).

Eglash, Plane, and Mundt (2006) describe a collection of physical and laboratory findings in a population of mothers with nipple lesions, deep breast aching or pain, and tender breasts upon palpation. Half of the mothers' nipples showed positive cultures for pathogenic bacteria and 75% had nipple cracks, blisters, or yellow scabs. The presence of nipple cracks was thought to be a vector for a bacterial lactiferous duct infection that responded to an average of five weeks of antibiotic treatment.

Eglash and Proctor (2007) describe a mother with a prolonged history of nipple cracks; dull throbbing of the breasts; sharp, shooting pains; pain on palpation of the breasts; and redness and swelling of the left breast. The chronic nipple sores did not heal in spite of systemic treatment with clindamycin. Laboratory findings of the cultured milk showed viridans *Streptococcus* and coagulase negative *Staphylococcus*. The authors postulate that the clinical and laboratory findings were descriptive of infections caused by small colony variants (SCVs) of staphylococci.

***Staphylococcus aureus* small colony variants** (SCVs) are a subpopulation of bacteria, which are implicated in recurrent and antibiotic refractory infections, probably due to their ability to evade the host immune defense (Proctor et al., 2006). SCVs cause low grade, persistent, antibiotic resistant, chronic and recurrent infections that take many weeks of antibiotics to clear (von Eiff, Peters, & Becker, 2006). This type of bacterial infection is resistant to aminoglycosides and may respond better to macrolides for a four-to-eight week duration. If a nipple infection persists in spite of topical or systemic antibiotic therapy, clinicians may wish to consider laboratory testing for SCVs.

Symptoms of Mastitis

Clinicians should be vigilant for an ascending infection when a mother presents with severe nipple pain or a break of any sort in the nipple skin because there is a significantly increased risk for mastitis in the presence of cracked nipples (Kinlay, O'Connell, & Kinlay, 2001). Open nipple lesions have a close association with mastitis, and both clinicians and mothers should not delay in starting treatment of these wounds (Fetherston, 1998;

Foxman, D'Arcy, Gillespie, Bobo, & Schwartz, 2002; Osterman & Rahm, 2000). In a study of 28 mothers with nipple pain, 57% had nipple swabs positive for *S. aureus* and 48% had positive milk specimens, indicative of ascending infection of the lactiferous ducts (Graves, Wright, Harman, & Bailey, 2003). Mothers complaining of deep breast pain are frequently treated for fungal infections; however, Thomassen, Johansson, Wassberg, and Petrini (1998) found that bacteria were often found both on the nipple and in the milk of mothers who described deep breast pain during or after breastfeeding.

Stages of Wound Healing

Wound healing is a complex process. There are partial thickness wounds with tissue destruction involving the epidermis and extending to, but not through, the dermis, and there are full thickness wounds that extend through the dermis and beyond (**Figure 2-2**).

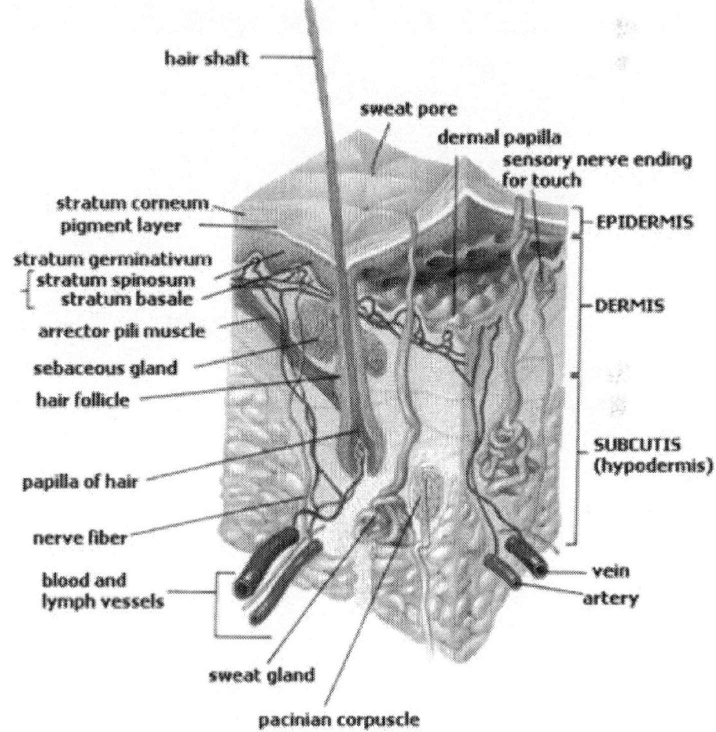

Figure 2-2. Cross Section of the Skin
From http://simple.wikipedia.org/wiki/File:Skin.jpg. Originally published by the National Cancer Institute in SEER Melanoma Training Module.

Mohrbacher (2010) has proposed a nipple trauma classification system to help provide consistency in the description of nipple damage:

Stage I: Superficial pain, intact skin, may see erythema (redness), bruising, edema

Stage II: Superficial pain, some tissue breakdown (abrasion, shallow fissure, compression stripe, blistering)

Stage III: Partial thickness erosion (skin breakdown to the lower layers of the dermis; deep fissure)

Stage IV: Full thickness erosion (full erosion through the dermis)

Winter (1962) described wound healing under moist conditions, but it is relatively recently that this concept was borrowed from the wound management knowledge base and applied to healing damaged nipples. As described earlier, moist wound healing has a number of advantages over dry wound healing. Wound repair involves the activity of a host of different cells which cannot function in a dry environment. The creation of new blood vessels occurs toward regions of low oxygen tension such that a wound covered by an occlusive dressing may stimulate this process. Debridement of the wound is enhanced in a moist environment. In larger or deeper wounds, epidermal cells must spread over the wound surface from the edges, and they require a supply of blood and nutrients.

Dry, crusted wounds reduce the blood and nutrient supply and pose a barrier to cell migration, which slows wound closure. A moist environment provided by an occlusive or semi-occlusive dressing poses a barrier to bacterial migration into the wound and insulates nerve endings to reduce pain. Turner (1979) discussed that the ideal dressing should have seven characteristics: remove excess exudate and toxins, provide high humidity at the interface between wound and dressing, allow for gas exchange, provide thermal insulation, protect against a secondary infection, be free from particulate and toxic components, and offer no trauma with removal.

Hydrogel Dressings

Because they are mostly composed of water, hydrogel dressings cool the wound, providing a measure of comfort during the healing process. Hydrogel dressings are generally combinations of water or glycerin in a polymer matrix. In the U.S., the Food and Drug Administration has designed hydrogel dressings as Class-I devices, which means they have minimal regulation. Moist dressings have been shown to decrease the days to complete healing, with subjects reporting reduced pain scores compared with dry-wound-healing methods (Wiechula 2003).

When observing treatment methods for wound healing on other parts of the body, occlusive or semiocclusive dressings are frequently used to cover the wound, maintain moisture, inhibit scab or crust formation, reduce pain, and enhance epithelial migration for wound repair (Ziemer, Cooper, & Pigeon, 1995). These authors studied the prophylactic use of a polyethylene film dressing (BlisterFilm, Sherwood Medical) with an adhesive border on the occurrence of nipple skin damage during the first week of breastfeeding. Although significantly reducing pain, this dressing did not prevent skin changes and damage. A high drop-out rate was seen due to skin pain and damage from the adhesive backing when the dressing was removed. No special breastfeeding instructions or corrections of feeding mechanics were provided for the mothers.

Building on the approach of using occlusive wound dressings for healing damaged nipples, Brent et al. (1998) randomized 42 mothers to receive a hydrogel wound dressing or a combination of breast shells and lanolin. The hydrogel dressing (Elasto-gel, Southwest Technologies, Inc.) was glycerin-based, highly absorbent, and non-adhesive, with cooling properties. Breastfeeding technique was controlled for and help provided when needed. Mothers using the breast shells and lanolin experienced fewer breast infections and less pain than the group using the glycerin-based dressing. Cable, Stewart, and Davis (1997) used a water-based hydrogel dressing (ClearSite, New Dimensions in Medicine/ConMed) to avoid potential problems with breast infections associated with glycerin-based products. Mothers in their study experienced significant pain relief when the dressing was worn between feedings. The sheet was changed every one to three days until the nipple wound healed.

Dodd and Chalmers (2003) compared the prophylactic use of lanolin with the water-based hydrogel dressing MaterniMates (Tyco Healthcare Group; currently marketed as Ameda ComfortGel, Ameda, Inc.). Mothers reported significantly lower pain scores when using the hydrogel dressing as a preventive measure, with no breast infections (versus eight cases of mastitis in the lanolin group).

Cadwell and colleagues (2004) studied the use of a glycerin-based hydrogel dressing (Soothies, Puronyx, Inc.) versus lanolin-application/breast-shell use versus breastfeeding education and support for mothers presenting with established nipple pain and damage. Rates of healing between the three groups were similar, but the mothers using the hydrogel pads experienced more relief from pain than the lanolin/shell group. Benbow and Vardy-White (2004) compared the use of Mothermates (Tyco Healthcare group) with traditional education and breastmilk applied to the nipple. Hydrogel dressings provided comfort to mothers, but a large difference was not seen between the two groups. The moist-wound healing options of lanolin and hydrogel dressings have been used both prophylactically to prevent nipple pain and damage, and therapeutically as remedies.

Lanolin may be a reasonable choice for sore or abraded nipples (Stage I and Stage II), while a hydrogel dressing may prove helpful for open sores or cracks with exudate (Stage III and Stage IV). The dressing absorbs wound discharge and prevents the skin from adhering to the mother's bra. Wound healing may be delayed in mothers who have diabetes or who are anemic. Clinicians should choose a hydrogel dressing that does not require adhesives to stick to the breast. Mothers have complained that some brands of hydrogel are very sticky, providing a further irritant to the nipples when removed. When taken off for feedings, hydrogels should not leave any residues or small pieces that adhere to the nipples. A sample intervention plan appears in **Box 2-7**.

Box 2-7. Sample Intervention Plans for Cracked/Damaged Nipples

Correct positioning and latch.

If there is a break in the nipple skin:

- Wash nipple with soap and water once each day.
- Apply topical mupirocin.
- Avoid pacifier use or wash pacifiers thoroughly with soap and water.
- Apply topical low strength steroids for inflammation.

If exudate is seen, erythema increases, or dry scab is present:

- Add systemic antibiotics.

If *Candida albicans* is suspected, add 2% miconazole.

If infection is recurrent or persistent:

- Treat infant with nasal mupirocin.
- Test for SCV, ask for culture and sensitivity laboratory testing.

If SCV are present switch to macrolide therapy;

- Use hydrogel dressing for comfort and moist wound healing.
- Be watchful for an ascending infection (mastitis).
- Correct anemia.

Other Possible Causes of Nipple Pain

Persistence or worsening of nipple pain requires careful history taking and direct observation to identify the cause (Walker & Driscoll, 1989). Assessing and treating sore or damaged nipples is difficult by telephone and may not capture the etiology of the problem. Women with nipple pain and cracked nipples report higher stress levels and abandon breastfeeding sooner than mothers without this problem (Abou-Dakn, Schafer-Graf, & Wockel, 2009). Mothers in distress from sore or cracked nipples need immediate measures for relief and remediation of this problem. It is also important to assess nipples for other possible causes of nipple pain, which can include the following.

Eczema: Eczema is a general term for several types of dermatitis, including atopic, seborrhea, irritant contact, and allergic contact, which usually respond to removing the irritant or allergen and/or the application of topical corticosteroids (Amir, 1993). Eczema can be present on the nipple itself or can extend onto and beyond the areola, with approximately half of the breastfeeding women who develop nipple and areolar eczema having a prior history of eczema (Barankin & Gross, 2004). Some mothers will develop eczema as a contact dermatitis following the introduction of solid foods into the infant's diet.

The clinical appearance can include erythema, papules, vesicles (fluid-filled blisters), oozing (Rago, 1988), crusts, lichenification (thickening and hardening of the skin), skin erosion, fissures, excoriations, and scaling (Ward & Burton, 1997). Burning and/or itching are typical symptoms of eczema (Bracket, 1988). Differentially, itching is not prominent in candidal infections and mammary candidiasis does not spare the area of the areola immediately adjacent to the nipple (Barankin & Gross, 2004).

Irritant contact dermatitis can be caused by soap, detergent, fragrances, or ointments. Offending agents in allergic contact dermatitis can include chamomile, vitamins A and E, aloe vera, perfumes, lanolin, and preservatives in some preparations of mycostatin formulations (Barankin & Gross, 2004). Topical corticosteroids are typically used in treating most episodes of eczema. The medication is applied to the affected areas after the infant has fed. The ointment should be wiped off prior to feedings, which can be done by expressing a small amount of milk onto the nipple and using this to wash off the medication.

In many instances, atopic dermatitis is accompanied by high colony counts of *S. aureus*, necessitating treatment with a topical antibiotic (Lever et al., 1988). This is especially true if there are also cracks on the nipple. If the eczema has appeared after introducing solid foods, the mother can be advised to rinse the nipple and areola with her expressed milk or with water and pat dry following feedings. Both nipples are commonly involved.

When eczema appears on just one nipple, the clinician should consider referral to rule out the presence of Paget's disease, which has the appearance of a steadily progressing eczema. Paget's disease of the nipple is a superficial manifestation of an underlying breast malignancy, thought to account for 1% to 3% of all breast cancers (Osther, Balsley, & Blichert-Toft, 1990). The lesion appears as a well-demarcated, red, scaly plaque appearing on the nipple first and then spreading to the areola. Oozing, crusting, itching, burning, skin thickening, erythema, ulceration, and nipple retraction may be present superficially, with a 60% occurrence of an underlying breast mass. A small vesicular eruption on the nipple, persistent soreness, pain, or itching of the nipple/areolar complex in the absence of other clinical symptoms may be the early manifestations of this condition (Jamali, Ricci, & Deckers, 1996). A biopsy establishes the diagnosis. Psoriasis can also involve the nipple with changes that include excoriation and ulceration (Islam, Karimeddini, Spencer Kurtzman, & Vento, 2000).

Herpes infection: Numerous discrete lesions at the junction of the nipple and areola and/or farther back on the areola can be a herpes simplex infection (Amir, 2004). The mother usually has extreme pain, and cultures of the lesions generally show herpes simplex type 1. Herpes in the neonate can be serious or fatal, and it can be transmitted through direct contact with active lesions (Sullivan-Bolyai et al., 1983). The mother can continue to breastfeed on the non-affected side, resuming on the infected side when the lesions have fully healed (American Academy of Pediatrics, 2005).

Herpes can infect intact skin (Dekio, Kawasaki, & Jidoi et al., 1986) and can originate in the baby's mouth from gingivostomatitis (Sealander & Kerr, 1989), a condition peaking in children between six months and three years of age. Infants with this condition can infect the maternal breast with herpes (Sealander & Kerr, 1989). Older infants and toddlers with sores in the anterior portion of the mouth and who refuse to eat should be checked for this condition. Mothers should take extra care in washing their hands if they, their older child, or their infant have herpes.

Raynaud's phenomenon of the nipple: Raynaud's phenomenon was first described in 1862 as intermittent ischemia typically affecting the fingers and toes, but it can involve other parts of the body, including blood vessels supplying the heart, gastrointestinal system, genitourinary system, and placental vasculature. This phenomenon can also affect the ear lobes, lips, nose, and nipples (Reilly & Snyder, 2005). It is more common in women than men, affecting up to 20% of women in the 21 to 50 year age group (Olsen & Nielson, 1978). Aggravating factors include exposure to cold, emotional stress (Morino & Winn, 2007), smoking, alcohol use, caffeine intake, and certain medications.

Raynaud's is associated with migraine headaches, as both conditions share a common vasospastic mechanism. In susceptible people and those with autoimmune diseases, such as lupus, rheumatoid arthritis, and systemic sclerosis, a precipitating event, such as exposure to cold temperatures, causes vasospasms of arterioles and intermittent ischemia to the affected body part. With breastfeeding, Raynaud's of the nipples usually occurs directly after the infant comes off the breast and the nipple is exposed to air that is cooler than the infant's mouth. Clinically, this is seen as pallor or blanching, followed by a cyanotic coloring as oxygen is cut off from the venous blood, ending with erythema (redness) as reflex vasodilation occurs. These color changes may involve all three changes (triphasic) or just two changes (biphasic). It is felt as a sensation of pain, burning, numbness, prickling, or stinging.

Gunther (1970) described this type of vasospasm in the nipple, but attributed it to psychosomatic causes. This is not entirely incorrect since psychological stress can trigger symptoms. But there are often underlying physical causes as well. Coates (1992) described bilateral nipple vasospasms in a mother who complained of intense pain, biphasic color changes, and partial relief from heat applications to the nipples. Because heat provided some relief and the symptoms were bilateral, it was suggested that this particular set of conditions could be a variant of Raynaud's phenomenon. Blanching of the nipples can occur not only during or just following a feeding, but also between feedings, with or without a history of Raynaud's in other parts of the body, and in conjunction with nipple trauma, such as ulceration, cracking, or blistering (Lawlor-Smith & Lawlor-Smith, 1997).

The pain associated with nipple vasospasm can be so throbbing and severe that some women may completely abandon breastfeeding. It can also occur with subsequent pregnancies. Other causes of nipple blanching and pain arise from inappropriate positioning, faulty latching, and variations of infant sucking that cause mechanical trauma from biting the nipple. A diagnosis of Raynaud's requires that other factors be present, such as the biphasic or triphasic color changes and precipitation by a stimulus, such as cold temperatures. Because of the nature of the pain, Raynaud's of the nipples may be misidentified as a *C. albicans* infection and treated with medications that provide no relief from the symptoms.

Many of the options for treating this condition are extrapolated from interventions used for Raynaud's phenomenon occurring in other parts of the body. The provision of warmth and the avoidance of cold stress are the first-line management options for Raynaud's of the nipples (Lawlor-Smith & Lawlor-Smith, 1996). Mothers may need to keep their entire body warm, use a heating pad over the breasts, wear warm clothing, wear warm coverings over the breasts, sleep under an electric blanket, or have warm packs available for application to the breast not being nursed on. If vasospasms occur between feedings, some mothers find relief by immersing the breasts in warm water.

Mothers with Raynaud's should avoid vasoconstricting drugs, such as caffeine and nicotine. Mothers experiencing this acute pain during lactation require immediate relief if breastfeeding is to continue. Nifedipine, a calcium channel blocker with vasodilating effects, has been used successfully to treat Raynaud's of the nipples (Anderson, Held, & Wright, 2004; Page & McKenna, 2006). Only small amounts are measurable in breastmilk (Ehrenkranz, Ackerman, & Hulse, 1989; Hale, 2008) and the American Academy of Pediatrics (2001) identifies the drug as usually compatible with breastfeeding. Nifedipine can be prescribed for dosing as 5 mg three times per day or as 30–60 mg per day in slow-release formulations. Usually one two-week course eliminates the symptoms, but some mothers may require two or three courses of treatment for complete resolution (Garrison, 2002).

Nipple bleb: A nipple bleb typically represents a nipple pore that is blocked by milk seeping under the epidermis causing a raised, opaque, shiny, white bump on the tip of the nipple. The mother usually complains of extreme pinpoint pain when the baby feeds. The incidence is unknown and speculation on its cause has mentioned a tendency in some people for epithelial overgrowth or the encouragement of epithelial growth by the epithelial growth factor in the mother's milk (Noble, 1991). If this tissue overgrowth obstructs milk flow from a nipple pore that drains a larger area of the breast, the possibility exists for milk stasis, a plugged duct farther back in the breast, or mastitis.

If the bleb does not open spontaneously, some mothers soften the skin with warm saline soaks, olive oil, and gentle rubbing with a towel or scraping with sterilized tweezers. If these efforts are unsuccessful, the mother's healthcare provider can open it with a sterile needle and express out any material that has accumulated behind it. Some of this material may be thick and stringy, representing milk that has thickened as the water in it is reabsorbed by the body. Many mothers who experience continuous nipple blebs learn to open them at home.

Anecdotal reports of successful resolution of a blocked nipple pore have been reported with the use of lecithin rubbed into the nipple following each feeding. Lecithin is a food additive used as an emulsifier that keeps fats from clumping together. Whereas a nipple bleb presents on the face of the nipple, a sebaceous cyst has been reported on the shaft or side of the nipple, with relief obtained when the oily material was removed (Wilson-Clay & Hoover, 2008). Not all white spots on the tip of the nipple are associated with a blocked nipple pore. Lawrence and Lawrence (2005) speculate that some white spots may be a buildup of cells similar to seborrheic dermatitis or cradle cap against which topical lecithin may be effective.

Incorrect pump flange size: Wilson-Clay and Hoover (2008) have observed that nipples swell during pumping. Using a circle template, they took pre- and post-pumping measurements of the nipple, showing that it can increase in size by as much as 3 to 4 mm. As a comparison, the pre-pumping nipple was about the size of a U.S. nickel, while after pumping the nipple was about the size of a U.S. quarter. Meier, Motyhowski, and Zuleger (2004) observed a sample of 35 mothers expressing milk for their preterm infants. As lactation progressed, about one-half of these mothers required a flange size that was larger than the standard flange that came with the pump's milk collection kit. Standard flange size is 23-24 mm, i.e., the diameter of the opening through which the nipple protrudes into the nipple or flange tunnel. As the study progressed, 77% of the mothers found that they required a larger flange, 27-30 mm, to remain free of pain and to express the maximum amount of milk. Flanges that are too small can contribute to nipple pain and cracks at the base of the nipple. A poor fit between nipple and flange reduces or eliminates the space between the nipple and the inner walls of the flange, potentially compromising the amount of milk that can be expressed because air movement is restricted and contributing to nipple pain.

A properly fitted flange demonstrates space between the nipple and the inner walls, as the nipple moves freely back and forth during pumping (**Figure 2-3**). Residual milk that is not removed will gradually contribute to down regulation of the milk supply and provide the potential for plugged milk ducts, focal points of engorgement, and mastitis.

Figure 2-3. Poor and Good Fits of Breast Pump Flanges

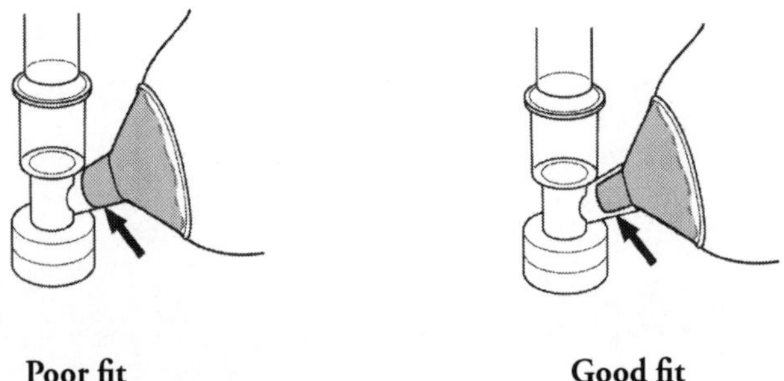

Poor fit **Good fit**

©Ameda Breastfeeding Products, used with permission.

Jones, Dimmock, and Spencer (2001) found that almost one-third of the 36 women in their study of preterm pumping mothers experienced disparity in the fit between their nipple and the size of the pump flange's nipple tunnel. Pump flanges can also be too large, which can contribute to nipple pain and damage to the areola. Some mothers may find that they need a different size shield for each breast and/or that as lactation progresses they no longer need a larger size shield (Jones & Hilton, 2009). It can take some experimentation to find the correctly fitting shield. Fitting guidelines should take the following into account.

A mother may need a larger flange if:

- The nipple rubs against the side of the nipple tunnel or sticks to the side.
- The nipple does not move freely in the tunnel after about 5 minutes of pumping.
- All of the nipple does not fit into the nipple tunnel.
- The nipple does not move back and forth in a smooth rhythmical motion.
- The mother experiences nipple pain while pumping.
- The tip of the nipple becomes sore or blistered.
- There are areas of the breast that are not well drained after pumping.
- A ring of sloughed skin or specks of skin are seen on the inside of the shield after pumping.
- The base of the nipple is blanching (turning white) while pumping.
- There is minimal or no areolar tissue being pulled into the tunnel of the breastshield.

The mother may need a smaller flange if:

- The shield does not stay in complete contact with the skin or are there gaps that would compromise suction.

If the mother is pumping 5-8 times per day, she may find that applying nipple cream or olive oil to the nipple and areola prior to pumping makes for a better seal and prevents abrasion of the nipple.

Some mothers find that many of the standard flanges still do not give them the fit they require or that milk production is being compromised by an incompatible fit between breast and flange. Other mothers feel uncomfortable leaning forward or assuming uncomfortable positions to properly place the flanges. To help mothers achieve a proper fit, the Pumpin Pal shield is sometimes used as an insert into a standard pump flange. The Pumpin Pal is angled (**Figure 2-4**) and accommodates some nipples in a more comfortable and efficient manner. It also allows a mother to lean back while pumping and fits into most brands of pumps.

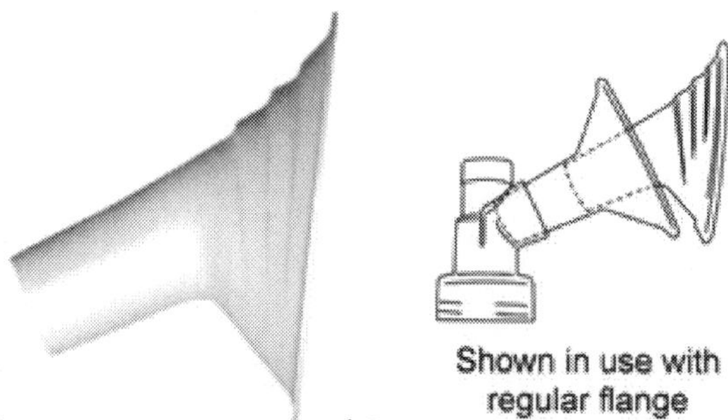

Figure 2-4. Pumpin' Pal Super Shield
Pumpin' Pal International, used with permission.

Mothers or clinicians can measure the nipple size at the base of the nipple. If the nipple is 20 mm in diameter or larger, she may wish to use one size larger than the standard flange. Many manufacturers provide a number of different size flanges (**Table 2-3**). Some clinicians with access to autoclaving or similar sterilizing facilities offer mothers the option of trying several different size flanges for an optimal fit.

Table 2-3. Breast Pump Flange Sizes

Manufacturer	Flange	Tunnel diameter
Ameda	Extra small insert	21.0 mm
	Small insert	22.5 mm
	Standard	25.0 mm
	Medium	28.5 mm
	Large	30.5 mm
	XL	32.5 mm
	XXL	36.0 mm
Medela	Small	21.0 mm
	Standard (Medium)	24.0 mm
	Large	27.0 mm
	XL	30.0 mm
	XXL	36.0 mm
	Blown glass	40.0 mm
Pumpin Pal	Original	23-29 mm
	Large	29-35 mm
	XL	35 mm+
Hygeia	Standard	27.0 mm
Avent	Standard	27.0 mm
	Insert	24.0 mm

Hyperkeratosis

Nevoid hyperkeratosis of the nipple and areola (NHNA) is a rare condition in which the skin of the nipple and/or areola becomes diffusely thickened, hyperpigmented, and covered with papules or hyperpigmented plaques. The lesions may be unilateral or bilateral. They may involve the nipple, areola, or both. The lesions are generally asymptomatic, but occasionally they may be itchy. Difficulty in breastfeeding has been reported (Perez-Izquierdo et al, 1990; Shastry, Betkerur, & Kushalappa, 2006). The etiology of NHNA is not known. A change in estrogen levels has been thought to precipitate this condition since it often worsens during pregnancy. Prolonged friction and rubbing of the nipple can induce thickening and hyperkeratosis (jogger's or cyclist's nipple), which can mimic NHNA. Topical preparations are usually applied to improve this condition.

Fungal Colonization

In addition to mechanical trauma of the nipple and bacterial infection, the fungal pathogen *C. albicans* can contribute to nipple and breast pain in lactating women. *C. albicans* is an opportunistic, commensal, normally harmless organism residing on the skin and in the gastrointestinal and genitourinary tracts. Dry, healthy, intact skin and the presence of normal competing flora typically allow *C. albicans* to exist in harmony with its host.

C. albicans exists in at least three different morphologies (forms): yeast, pseudohyphae, and hyphae. By activating appropriate sets of genes, it can alter its form to adapt to its changing environment and increase its virulence, allowing it to colonize or infect virtually all body sites (Staib et al., 2000). *C. albicans* may appear as spherical yeast cells on the skin, and while they can change into filamentous forms that readily penetrate tissues, the organism has many other mechanisms to circumvent and take advantage of changing host conditions. The filamentous forms of hyphae and pseudohyphae adhere better to epithelial cells than spherical yeast cells. Their projections can follow surface discontinuities and penetrate through breaks in tissue, such as those occurring in nipple fissures (Odds, 1994). They can secrete enzymes that digest epidermal keratin, the tough top layer of skin, assisting hyphal filaments in their invasive process and inducing an inflammatory response.

Risk factors for mammary candidosis:

- Between 22% (Cotch, Hillier, Gibbs, & Eschenbach, 1998) and 33% (Vidotto et al., 1992) of pregnant women test positive for vaginal candidosis by the end of their pregnancy, with the majority (95%) caused by *C. albicans* (Odds, 1994).
- Use of antibiotics or steroids during the peripartum period or while breastfeeding increases the risk (Amir, Garland, Dennerstein, & Farish, 1996; Chetwynd, Ives, Payne, & Edens-Bartholomew, 2002; Dinsmoor, Viloria, Lief, & Elder, 2005; Tanquay, McBean, & Jain, 1994).
- Mothers with diabetes or a history of polycystic ovary syndrome are prone to candida overgrowth as candida thrives in a sugar-rich environment. Hyperglycemic individuals may have an increased

risk for candida colonization because their secretions contain glucose, which can serve as nutrients for candida organisms.

- Sore or damaged nipples provide a route of entry for pathogens (Amir, 1991; Amir et al., 1996; Amir & Hoover, 2003; Livingstone et al., 1996; Tanquay et al., 1994).
- Colonization and development of oral thrush occur in infants from the birth process (Remington & Klein, 1983) and other vectors, such as healthcare workers (Pfaller, 1994), as the infant gets older. Forty percent to 60% of infants carry the organism in their mouths, with 10% to 24% developing oral thrush within the first 18 months (Darwazeh & al-Bashir, 1995). Morrill, Heinig, Pappagianis, and Dewey (2005) reported oral colonization in 20% of infants studied, of whom 75% developed oral thrush by nine weeks of age.
- Use of pacifiers in infants (Brook & Gober, 1997; Darwazeh & al-Bashir, 1995; Mattos-Graner, de Moraes, Rontani, & Birman, 2001) may not only facilitate oral colonization, but contribute to persistence of candidal presence in the mouth (Manning, Coughlin, & Poskitt, 1985). Candida species have the ability to form biofilms to protect their colonies, just as bacteria can. The tenacious grip of *C. albicans* on pacifiers and their plastic mouth shields was shown in a study that measured biofilm growth on latex and silicone pacifiers. Biofilm formation developed on both latex and silicone pacifiers and their plastic mouth shields, with silicone being slightly more resistant to fungal colonization due to its smoother surface (da Silveira, Charone, Maia, Soares, & Portela, 2009). In mixed species biofilms of candida and staphylococcus, the organisms can work synergistically to prevent the penetration of antibacterials and antifungals in the treatment of the infection. Adam, Baillie, and Douglas (2002) showed that in mixed fungal-bacterial biofilms, the fungal cells could modulate the action of antibiotics and bacteria could affect antifungal activity. This may be a contributor to the difficulty seen in eradicating some persistent fungal infections. Failure to sufficiently clean pacifiers of infants with fungal colonization in the mouth may lead to reinfection of the mother's nipples each time such a pacifier is used.
- The use of bottles has been demonstrated to be a key risk factor for *C. albicans* colonization in both mothers and infants. Morrill et al. (2005) reported that of 52 mother/baby dyads that used bottles in the first two weeks postpartum, 44% of the mothers and 38% of the infants tested positive for *C. albicans*. They suggest

> that it may not be bottle use alone, but the fluid contained in the bottle that provides the growth medium for facilitating *C. albicans* colonization. Infant formula contains large amounts of iron, with iron being known to increase growth of *C. albicans* in vitro (Andersson, Lindquist, Lagerqvust, & Hernell, 2000). Lactoferrin in human milk typically keeps *C. albicans* in check. However, the absence of lactoferrin in artificial baby milks, plus its relatively heavy load of iron may combine to augment yeast proliferation in the infant's mouth. *C. albicans* adherence to epithelial surfaces can also be encouraged by the presence of sucrose or fructose (Pizzo, Giuliana, Milici, & Giangreco, 2000), such as seen in soy-based infant formulas. Some soy-based formulas can contain as much as 10% sucrose (table sugar). Thus mothers who supplement breastfeeding with bottles of infant formula, especially certain soy formulas, are at increased risk of contracting a fungal nipple infection from the mouth of their infant.

The exact prevalence of *C. albicans* colonization in mothers is not known. Twenty-six percent of breastfeeding women referred to a clinic for nipple and breast pain fulfilled the clinical diagnosis for nipple candidosis (Tanquay et al., 1994). Thomassen et al. (1998) reported that 50% of women with superficial nipple pain and 20% of women with deep breast pain had positive cultures for *C. albicans*. Thus, deep breast pain or shooting breast pain by itself may not be indicative of candidal infection within the breast (Carmichael & Dixon, 2002).

In a healthy population of lactating women, Morrill et al. (2005) found that 23% were colonized by candida species on the nipple/areola or in their milk. The occurrence of mammary candidosis, defined as colonization plus symptoms, was 20% between two and nine weeks postpartum. In the Morrill study, the rate of weaning by nine weeks for this painful condition was 2.2 times higher in women who developed mammary candidosis. *C. albicans* was found more frequently in mothers who reported breastfeeding associated pain (Andrews et al., 2007), possibly due to nipple alterations that predispose to candidal overgrowth.

Not all candida species found on the nipple are *C. albicans*. Zollner and Jorge (2003) found several different strains of candida on the nipples and in the mouths of breastfeeding mothers and infants. However, in the bottle-feeding comparison group in this study, the prevalence of candida on the non-lactating breast was significantly lower. Breastfeeding can predispose the nipple to candida colonization. A prevalence of 34.55% for candida species was found in the mouths of breastfed infants who did not use pacifiers or artificial nipples and 66.67% in the mouths of infants who were exclusively bottle-fed. Hoppe (1997) considers both feeding bottles and pacifiers as vectors for the transmission of candida. In a mother/baby pair at increased risk for candida infection, use of pacifiers and artificial nipples should be discouraged.

Detecting *C. albicans* and diagnosing mammary candidosis can be difficult, especially since other nipple and breast discomforts share some similar symptoms (Wiener, 2006). Accurate detection of candidal species in human milk is complicated by the action of lactoferrin. The lactoferrin in human milk inhibits yeast growth in vitro (Soukka, Tenovuo, & Lenander-Lemikari, 1992), often resulting in false-negative test results when the milk is cultured. Skin scrapings of the nipple/areola can be placed under a microscope in a 10% KOH (potassium hydroxide) wet mount to identify the presence of yeast, yet few clinicians order any type of laboratory testing to identify and diagnose mammary candidosis (Brent, 2001).

A laboratory technique that uses the addition of iron to counteract the action of lactoferrin has been shown to reduce the likelihood of false-negative test results and provide a more accurate means of confirming the presence of candida in human milk (Morrill et al., 2003). Accurate laboratory testing still takes about three days, leaving the mother in pain and validating the need for a more rapid means of determining when and how to treat the symptoms.

Mammary candidosis is most often diagnosed presumptively by signs and symptoms that are subjective, can be indicative of other problems, and are rarely confirmed by laboratory findings (Amir & Pakula, 1991; Johnstone & Marcinak, 1990). Signs include a nipple and/or areola that is red, shiny, or flaky. Symptoms include burning pain of the nipple/areola and deep, shooting, burning, or stabbing pain in the breast. In an effort to better delineate the signs and symptoms clinicians could use to determine treatment, Morrill et al. (2004) used the measure of positive predictive value (PPV) for each sign and symptom. PPV was chosen as a measure because a PPV value above 70% is considered to be of clinical value (Grimes & Schulz, 2002). The PPV value was 50% or less for each of the signs and symptoms when they occurred individually. Thus, burning or stabbing sensations by themselves are not necessarily indicative of candida and may not warrant fungal treatment. However, when certain combinations of signs and symptoms occurred, the PPV rose to over 70% (**Table 2-4**), indicating that there was a high probability that the mother had candida. The high probability combinations are:

- When the signs of shiny and flaky skin of the nipple/areola occur together.
- When either of the skin symptoms occur, together with nonstabbing or stabbing breast pain.
- When combinations of three or more signs and symptoms occur simultaneously, especially when the combination includes either shiny or flaky skin of the nipple/areola.

Table 2-4. Positive Predictive Values of Signs and Symptoms of Candida on the Nipple

Signs and Symptoms	Positive Predictive Value (%)
Sore + burning + pain + stabbing + skin changes	100
Burning + pain + stabbing + skin changes	100
Pain + stabbing + skin changes	100
Sore + burning + pain + skin changes	80-91
Burning + pain + skin changes	80-85
Sore + burning + pain + stabbing	74
Burning + pain + stabbing	63
Pain + stabbing	57

Definitions used in this table:

Sore = sore but not burning nipple

Burning = burning pain on the nipple/areola

Pain = non-stabbing pain of the breast

Stabbing = stabbing pain in the breast

Skin changes = shiny skin on the nipple and/or flaky skin on the nipple/areola

Adapted from (Morrill et al., 2004 and Wiener, 2006).

Treatment approaches should begin by assessing and correcting mechanical causes of nipple pain, including assessing for Raynaud's syndrome of the nipples (Amir, 2003), because burning symptoms of the nipples alone may not be indicative of candida. If nipple pain persists following correction of breastfeeding techniques, bacterial infection may be present and can be treated with a topical antibiotic, such as mupirocin (Bactroban). However, if the nipple pain worsens or is described as a combination of any of the factors with a PPV above 70%, a combined bacterial and fungal infection may be present to which a topical antifungal, such as miconazole 2%, can be added.

For treating a suspected combined fungal and bacterial infection, Newman's all-purpose nipple ointment, part of the Newman Candida protocol (Newman & Kernerman, 2008) can be compounded in the following proportions:

- Mupirocin 2% ointment (15 grams)
- Betamethasone 0.1% ointment (15 grams)
- Miconazole powder is added so that the final concentration is 2% miconazole

Newman's ointment should be applied sparingly after each feeding until the mother is pain-free, and then decrease the frequency over a week or two until the pain stops. If this topical treatment provides no pain relief in three to four days or if it is needed for longer than two to three weeks to keep pain free, then the nipple/areolar skin and the milk should be tested.

If Newman's ointment does not provide complete relief, then Gentian violet treatment can be added. Gentian violet, a strong purple dye that kills yeast on contact, can be painted on the nipples and areolae using a 0.5% to 1.0% strength aqueous solution for four to seven days. At a higher concentration or used for a prolonged periods of time, gentian violet has the potential for toxicity (Piatt & Bergeson, 1992). Therefore, a dilution of 0.25% to 0.5% can be used in the baby's mouth once daily for four to seven days to avoid oral mucosal ulceration (Utter, 1990; Utter, 1992). If the pain is gone after four days, the gentian violet should be stopped. If the pain is better, but not gone after four days, treatment can continue for seven days. If the pain is not better at all at four days, stop the gentian violet, continue with the ointment. After seven days, gentian violet treatment should be stopped. Newman's Candida Protocol suggests that if candida persists, then add grapefruit seed extract (GSE), whose active ingredient must be "citricidal" (a powerful compound extracted from organically grown grapefruit that inhibits growth of parasites, fungi, and bacteria). Application to the nipples should be followed by and used in conjunction with Newman's ointment. A diluted solution should be applied directly on the nipples (**Box 2-8**).

Box 2-8. Dilution for Grapefruit See Extract (GSE)

- Put 5-10 drops in 30 ml (1 ounce) of water and mix very well.
- Use cotton swabs to apply to both nipples and areolas *after* the feeding.
- Let dry a few seconds, and then apply an "all purpose nipple ointment."
- If also using Gentian Violet, do not use GSE on that particular feed, but use after all other feeds.
- Use until pain is gone, and then wean down slowly over a period of at least a week.
- If pain is *not* significantly improving after two to three days, increase the concentration by 5 drops per 30 ml (ounce) of water. Can continue increasing concentration until using 25 drops/ 30 ml of water.
- If flaking, drying, or whiteness appears on the skin, substitute pure olive oil for the ointment 1-3x/day and decrease the concentration of the GSE drops. If the flaking does not get better, stop the GSE drops.
- Laundry can be treated as well: add 15-20 drops in the rinse cycle of all wash loads.
- May be used in conjunction with oral GSE and probiotics.

From Dr. Jack Newman's Candida Protocol: www.drjacknewman.com/.

If the pain and candida have not resolved, then systemic treatment with GSE can be added (**Box 2-9**).

Box 2-9. Oral GSE and Probiotics

- Grapefruit seed extract (*not* grape seed extract, active ingredient must be "citricidal") tablets or capsules, 250 mg (usually 2 tablets) three or four times a day orally (taken by the mother). If preferred, the liquid extract can be taken orally, 10 drops in water three times per day (though this is not as effective). Oral GSE can be used before trying fluconazole, instead of fluconazole, or in addition to fluconazole in resistant cases.
- Probiotics: Acidophilus with bifidus (with FOS (fructo-oligosaccharides) is okay). The mother should take 1-2 capsules (strength of 10 billion cells) 2-3x/day. The probiotics should be taken at least one hour apart from oral GSE. Baby should be treated with Probiotics 2x/day for approximately seven days (Mother may wet her finger and roll it in probiotic powder (break open a capsule), and let baby suck on mother's finger right before a feeding).

From Dr. Jack Newman's Candida Protocol: www.drjacknewman.com/.

Fluconazole (Diflucan) is a systemic agent that may be used when the previous treatments fail or when laboratory results confirm the presence of candida in the milk. The loading dose is usually 400 mg followed by 100 mg twice daily for two weeks, until the mother is pain free for a week. It should be used in combination with Newman's topical nipple ointment because fluconazole can take several days to start working. Some persistent or mismanaged cases of candidiasis may require a longer course of fluconazole, not only for the mother (Bodley & Powers, 1997), but also for the infant (Chetwynd et al., 2002). Both mother and baby should be treated simultaneously, even if thrush is not visible in the infant's mouth (Johnstone & Marcinak, 1990).

If there is no relief after 14 to 21 days of fluconazole treatment, the deep breast pain may have a different cause, such as a bacterial infection. Recently, Hale, Bateman, Finkelman, and Berens (2009) used new laboratory techniques for the detection of *C. albicans* to determine the presence of yeast in milk samples from mothers exhibiting sore nipples, stabbing or burning pain that radiated to the axilla, and painful breastfeeding without a specific diagnosis. The laboratory technique detects a cellular wall component of yeast, which if present in milk would be indicative of ductal candidal involvement. There was no significant difference in the presence of cultured fungal cellular wall components between the control and symptomatic groups. These data suggest that *C. albicans* does not grow inside the milk ducts of the breast and that its presence in expressed breastmilk could be accounted for by fungal species on the nipple, placed there by its presence in the infant's mouth.

There is a high correlation between oral and diaper candidosis among infants of mothers with nipple candidiasis (Tanguay et al., 1994). Mothers with deep breast pain may also benefit from anti-inflammatory pain medications, such as ibuprofen.

Nystatin (Mycostatin) has long been used on both the nipples of the mother and the oral mucosa of the infant. Treatment for infants should occur simultaneously but not with oral nystatin. Hoppe and Hahn (1997) compared the clinical cure rates of nystatin and miconazole gel in 227 infants who were treated four times a day following feeds. After 12 days of treatment, the miconazole gel had a cure rate of 99% compared with only a 54% cure rate in those infants where nystatin had been used (**Table 2-5**).

Table 2-5. Comparison of Cure Rates between Miconazole Gel and Nystatin for Infant Oral Thrush

Day	Miconazole Gel	Nystatin Suspension
5	84.7%	21.2%
8	96.9%	37.6%
12	99.0%	54.1%

Nystatin's effectiveness has been reduced over time because almost 45% of candida strains are resistant to nystatin (Hale & Berens, 2002). *C. albicans* persistently adheres to buccal mucosa and is less affected by nystatin than other candida species (Ellepola, Panagoda, & Samaranayake, 1999). Nystatin is more fugistatic than fungicidal, thus it may reduce symptoms in some mothers and infants, but it can be ineffective in eradicating the infection. If gentian violet is used for the infant's mouth, it should be diluted to a 0.25% or 0.5% solution.

Some mothers take acidophilus supplements (1 tablet daily containing 40 million to 1 billion viable units) to help restore a balance of microorganisms in the body. Mothers may question if the milk they express during a yeast infection can be given to the baby later. Under susceptible conditions, this milk may have the potential to infect or re-infect because freezing does not kill yeast (Rosa et al., 1990), although lactoferrin may keep yeast levels low.

Panjaitan, Amir, Costs, Rudland, and Tabrizi (2008) demonstrated an association between candida infection and nipple pain, but identified other fungal species on sore nipples, raising the possibility that nipple pain/thrush could be due to the presence of fungal organisms other than *C. albicans.*

The best defense against *C. albicans* is healthy, intact skin and a robust immune system. Efforts should be made to assure correct latch by the infant and assessment of any nipple pain reported by the mother. The longer incorrect sucking patterns persist, the greater the chance for both bacterial and fungal overgrowth of damaged nipple tissue. Pacifiers and bottles containing infant formulas should be avoided. Persistent nipple soreness, fissured nipples that are slow to heal, and nipples with obvious dermatologic abnormalities must be addressed immediately. Clinicians may consider avoiding the use of nystatin because it often prolongs the amount of time until the mother finds relief from the pain of a candidal infection. Unresolved nipple pain may cause untimely weaning (Schwartz et al., 2002). Both mother and baby should be treated if one or the other shows signs of candidiasis (**Figure 2-5**).

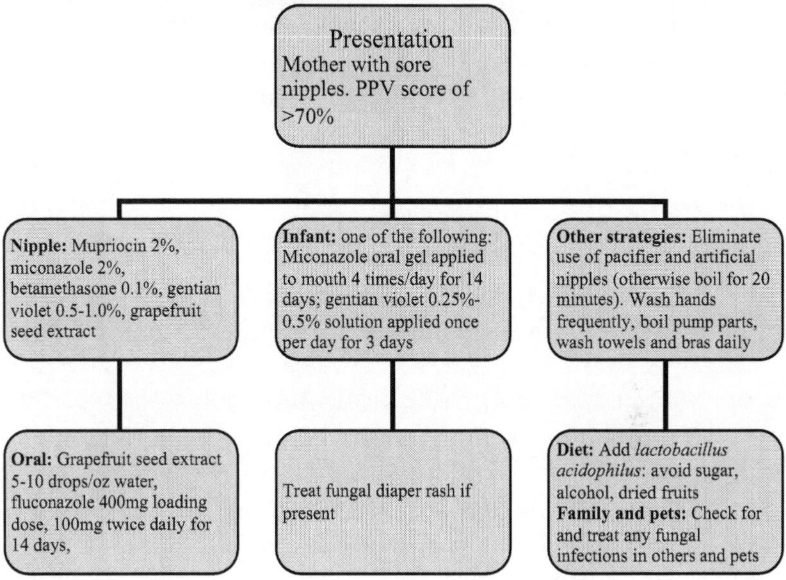

Figure 2-5. Sample Intervention Plan Flowchart for Candida

NIPPLE PIERCING

Nipple piercing has a long history, dating back to the 1300s and probably earlier. Women engage in intimate piercings for many reasons. They may believe that piercing makes the nipples larger, more sensitive, more sexually attractive, and may provide pleasure by the constant stimulation and erectness of the nipple. It was recommended by doctors in Victorian England to increase the size of the nipples to make breastfeeding easier.

In the months following this procedure, infection, mastitis, and abscess formation have been reported to be as high as 10–20%, with healing of the wound channel taking up to 6–12 months (Jacobs et al., 2003). Because some nipple piercings can take up to 18 months to heal or if there have been multiple piercings, the potential for scar tissue development can interfere with milk transfer, cause sore nipples, and/or contribute to plugged ducts and mastitis. If the piercing is less than one year old, it may not yet be fully healed, increasing the possibility of pain and infection.

Reputable professional piercers generally refuse to pierce the nipples of a pregnant woman. The piercing is generally through the body of the nipple at its base in a horizontal plane, although some piercings can be done in a vertical plane. Generally, women wear a horizontal or crescent shaped barbell or a captive bead (ring or hoop). Occasionally, the piercing is of an incorrect size or the jewelry is too small, causing migration of the jewelry into the nipple skin and generally resulting in pain and inflammation. Pregnancy usually does not affect the piercing (Armstrong, Caliendo, & Roberts, 2006). While most nipple piercings do not interfere with breastfeeding, awareness of potential problems is important:

- **Problems with latch.** Problems with infant latch may occur if the nipple jewelry remains in place while nursing. Some infants may not be able to latch correctly to the nipple or may find that the jewelry is uncomfortable or abrasive in their mouth.
- **Potential swallowing.** There is the potential for the infant to swallow, choke, or aspirate jewelry parts should they become dislodged during vigorous sucking. Jones (1999) reported the uncoupling of barbell jewelry during nursing.
- **Reduced milk transfer.** Reduced milk transfer may occur if the piercing penetrated the central duct bundle of the nipple or if a nipple is numb due to nerve damage. Reduced milk production and slow weight gain is possible. Loss of sensation to the nipple can impede milk ejection. Garbin, Deacon, Rowan, Hartmann, and Geddes (2009) reported on several mothers presenting to their research group with pierced nipples and a poor milk supply on the affected breast. Under ultrasound examination, a marked reduction in blood flow to the affected breast was seen, as well as septa in milk ducts within the affected breast of one of the mothers. Duct obstruction seems to be a potential side effect of some nipple piercings, with a reduction in the amount of milk synthesized in the affected breast due to ineffective milk removal. In mothers with an abundant milk supply, this may go unnoticed as the opposite breast compensates for low milk production in the contralateral side. In mothers with marginal milk production, this situation could result in poor infant weight gain.
- **Sore nipples.** Sore nipples are possible if the piercing is not fully healed. Some nipples become very sensitive following piercing, so even though there may not be damage to the nipple it may remain painful.

Clinicians are reminded to check pierced nipples for numbness, discharge, hypersensitivity, healing, and scar tissue when mothers present with one or both nipples with piercings (Martin, 2004). Milk may also leak through the piercings. Infant weight gain should be monitored closely in the early weeks.

Women with pierced nipples may fear that the piercing will close if they must remove the jewelry during the entire time they are breastfeeding, or they may find that removing and reinserting the jewelry before and after breastfeedings is perceived as a barrier to continued nursing. Some mothers use what is called a retainer that can be easily removed and inserted throughout the day to preserve the patency of the piercing. Some mothers regret the piercing and seek to reverse it. A surgical procedure that excises the epithelial tunnel core can be performed with minimal damage to the surrounding tissue (Sadove & Clayman, 2008). However, the potential still exists for damage to any number of ducts that lead to the nipple surface.

NIPPLE DISCHARGE

Observation of a colored discharge from the nipple can be quite frightening to a mother. The most common cause of nipple discharge is a benign papilloma followed by duct ectasia (Hussain, Policarpio, & Vincent, 2006). Duct ectasia is an inflammatory process producing a sticky discharge of various colors and is more common in older women. Dilatation of the terminal ducts during pregnancy may start a process of the formation of an irritating lipid, which triggers an inflammatory response and the resulting nipple discharge. Most often, the discharge is dark green or black, appearing to be blood, but actually testing guaiac negative (stool is negative for occult blood) (Falkenberry, 2002). The discharge is more commonly multiductal, bilateral, and colored. Smoking may be associated with duct ectasia (Rahal, deFreitas-Junior, & Paulinelli, 2005). The nipple and areola may also be painful, burn, itch, and swell. Clinicians should be watchful for plugging of the nipple pores and the development of a mass in the breast.

Other common nipple discharges include the following:

- Green, yellow, brown, reddish brown, or gray discharges may be associated with manipulation of the nipple at the end of a pregnancy or in early lactation (O'Callaghan, 1981). Such manipulation may disrupt delicate blood vessels within the nipple.
- Purulent (pus) discharge may be seen with mastitis or an abscess.

- It is not unheard of for a mother's early milk to contain traces of blood. Approximately 15% of asymptomatic lactating mothers have blood in their early milk when cytologically tested (Lafreniere, 1990). Delicate capillary networks that are traumatized during the rapid cellular proliferation that takes place during pregnancy may result in early milk that is blood tinged (Kline & Lash, 1962).
- Intraductal papilloma is a common cause of blood in the milk. This is a tiny growth from the lining of a milk duct with a vascular component that protrudes into the lumen or duct channel and can bleed when disrupted by breastfeeding or breast pumping. Most women are not aware of these growths unless they see blood in their pumped milk or if their infant vomits blood-tinged milk. The bleeding usually stops spontaneously. If an infant vomits blood-tinged milk, clinicians need to determine the source of the blood. Testing for fetal or adult hemoglobin determines the origin of the blood. If the infant tolerates the milk, he or she can continue breastfeeding from the affected side. If the infant cannot tolerate the blood because it acts as an emetic, the mother can pump her breast until the milk is clear of blood, usually from three to seven days.

Parents also need to know that they may see black flecks in the infant's stool or the stool may at times be black or tarry, as any ingested blood passes through the infant's intestines. Bloody nipple discharge that persists or that is accompanied by a lump under the nipple that does not resolve with feeding must be evaluated by the mother's physician.

BREAST SURGERY INVOLVING THE NIPPLE/AREOLA

Surgery of any type that involves the nipple and/or the areola either as a primary site or in peripheral sites that could impact the nipple are cause for concern for both mothers and clinicians.

Breast Augmentation

During breast augmentation surgery, if the primary nerve that innervates the nipple/areolar complex is stretched, cut, or cauterized, then nipple sensation can be affected. If the nerve is stretched, sensation generally returns with no problems. If the nerve is cut, nipple sensation is not likely to return. If the nerve is cauterized, there is a chance that nipple sensation will return, depending on the extent of the cauterization. The risk of permanent nipple numbness from augmentation surgery is about 15%. Using an implant whose diameter is larger than the breast's diameter increases the risk of nipple numbness. Women who choose very large implants relative to their breast skin envelopes risk loss of nipple sensation (Mofid, Klatsky, Singh, & Nahabedian, 2006). Sensation in some nipples can take up to two years to return following augmentation surgery. The periareolar incision site is often associated with the highest risk of interference with breastfeeding.

In a retrospective study that compared lactation outcomes between augmented and non-augmented women, 64% of 42 augmented women experienced insufficient lactation compared with less than 7% of 42 non-augmented women (Hurst, 1996). Strom, Baldwin, Sigurdson, and Schusterman (1997) reported on breastfeeding outcomes of 28 women from a study on 292 cosmetic saline implant patients, 46 of whom had children after the procedure. Of the 28 women who breastfed, 11 reported problems and eight reported breastfeeding problems they perceived as being related to the implants. Seven of the eight women had implants placed through a periareolar incision. Nerves innervating the nipple and areola are best protected if resections at the base of the breast and skin incisions at the medial areolar border are avoided (Schlenz, Kuzbari, Gruber, & Holle, 2000).

Breast Reduction

Women have a number of reasons for seeking breast reduction surgery that include musculoskeletal stress from large, heavy breasts, pain, poor body image, and restrictions on physical activities. Older surgical techniques involving the "free nipple graft" technique or the complete removal of the nipple–areolar complex and reattachment often resulted in impaired or impossible lactation. Nipple sensation is usually greatly diminished in these women, but not necessarily absent (Ahmed & Kolhe, 2000). A number of newer surgical techniques preserve the attachment of the nipple/areola complex to underlying tissue, as well as improve the vascular supply to the nipple with less disruption of sensory nerves (Gonzalez et al., 1993; Hallock, 1992; Nahabedian & Mofid, 2002).

Certain types of reduction mammaplasty may result in less of a compromise to lactation (Ramirez, 2002), making it important to inform women before reduction surgery about the procedure's potential effect on lactation. Cruz and Korchin (2007) found that loss of nipple sensation occurred in 2% of women who had undergone reduction mammaplasty, no matter what type of pedicle was used during surgery. Because of the intermixing of adipose tissue and glandular tissue, breast reduction surgery cannot be accomplished by a simple removal of "fat deposits," as with liposuction (Nickell & Skelton, 2005). Preserving the glandular tissue within the first 30 mm of the nipple and using a surgical technique that keeps the pedicle supporting the nipple–areolar complex as thick as possible may maximize the potential for optimal milk production (Nickell & Skelton, 2005; Ramsay et al., 2005). If a woman has only five or six main milk ducts, removal or destruction of just a few of those central ducts could permanently impair the milk production potential of that breast (Ramsay et al., 2005).

Mothers who have had reduction surgery should be encouraged to breastfeed with proper infant follow-up. The breastfeeding practices of a series of postpartum women who had undergone prior reduction mammaplasty by means of an inferior pedicle approach were reported in a retrospective study by Brzozowski, Ziessen, Evans, and Hurst (2000), who also examined the factors that influenced the decision to breastfeed postoperatively. Successful breastfeeding was defined as the ability to feed for a duration equal to or greater than two weeks. Seventy-eight patients had children after their breast reduction surgery. Fifteen of the 78 patients (19.2%) breastfed exclusively, eight (10.3%) breastfed with formula supplementation, 14 (17.9%) had an unsuccessful breastfeeding attempt, and 41 (52.6%) did not attempt breastfeeding. Of the 41 patients not attempting to breastfeed, nine patients did so as a direct consequence of discouragement by a healthcare professional.

Of the 78 women who had children postoperatively, a total of 27 were discouraged from breastfeeding by medical professionals, with only 8 of the 27 (29.6%) subsequently attempting to do so, despite this recommendation. In comparison, 26 patients were encouraged to breastfeed; 19 (73.1%) of them did subsequently attempt breastfeeding. Postpartum breast engorgement and lactation was experienced by 31 of the 41 patients not attempting to breastfeed. Of these 31 patients, 19 believed they would have been able to breastfeed due to the extent of breast engorgement and lactation experienced. Studies examining successful lactation outcomes after breast reduction surgery show varying results, with approximately 50% reported as successfully breastfeeding, depending on the type of surgery performed (Brzozowski et al., 2000).

The studies typically define successful breastfeeding as breastfeeding (with or without supplementation) for two to three weeks (Cherchel, Azzam, & De May, 2007; Chiummariello et al., 2008; Cruz & Korchin, 2007). Using this definition of successful breastfeeding can be misleading to clinicians and mothers. "Successful" breastfeeding could be accomplished for two weeks when infant intake may be small. After that time, supplementation may be necessary for some infants.

Mothers should understand that 100% milk production may not always be possible, but should still be strongly encouraged to breastfeed. Loss of nipple sensation has the potential to interrupt the feedback from the nipple to the pituitary gland, resulting in potential milk production problems. A mother who cannot feel her nipple runs an increased risk of damage and trauma to the nipples, infection, and incorrect infant latch. Mothers and infants require close follow-up in the early weeks with frequent infant weight checks.

West and Hirsch (2008) noted that postsurgical mothers may experience breast pain and/or nipple blanching or vasospasm of the nipple. Blanching may be due to a blood supply interruption or nerve trauma to the nipple/areolar complex during the surgery, although the true cause is unknown. Because the nipple/areola complex may have assumed an alternative or rather shallow shape following surgery, some infants may have difficulty latching or may engage in a very shallow latch, which could result in pain and nipple blanching. Mothers may find some relief from this painful condition by compressing the areola and mechanically squeezing blood back into the nipple (West & Hirsch, 2008). Breast pain may be related to scar tissue formation from the surgical procedure. However, clinicians should rule out incorrect latch and fungal or bacterial infections of the breast before attributing sharp breast pains to scar formation.

Box 2-10 provides a sample intervention plan for mothers with breast augmentation or breast reduction.

Box 2-10. Sample Intervention Plan for Mothers with Breast Augmentation or Reduction

Mothers and infants should be assessed and followed closely in the early days and weeks to assure that infant weight gain is adequate, milk production is sufficient, and damage to nipples is minimized.

- Advise mothers that reduction or augmentation surgery has the potential to disrupt breastfeeding.
- Assess latch and correct if necessary.
- Use methods to evert the nipple prior to feedings if nipple inversion from breast surgery is present.
- Feed 8-12 times per 24 hours.
- Hand express or pump milk if infant does not latch or feeds poorly.
- Assure milk transfer.
    - Use alternate massage on each breast at each feeding to maximize milk intake (alternate massage involves massaging and compressing the breast during each pause between sucking bursts).
    - Compress the breast from above rather than squeezing from below the breast if the mother has implants. The sides of the breast should be compressed such that pressure is avoided on the implant to prevent implant rupture.
    - Perform pre- and post-feed weights to quantify milk intake and determine if supplementation is necessary.
- Pump after feedings following discharge if needed.
    - Enhance milk output with power pumping (with double collection kit, pump for 5-8 minutes until milk flow slows with first let-down, remove pump and start pumping again 20 minutes later, repeat a third time; another power pumping session can be done in the evening).
- Weigh infant every three days until adequate weight gain pattern is established.
    - Weigh infant the day after discharge to prevent excessive weight loss and high bilirubin levels.
- Use expressed milk if supplement is needed; expressed milk can be delivered through a tube feeding device at the breast to maximize breast stimulation. If sufficient breast milk is not available, supplement with infant formula.
- Check nipples for pain or trauma with corrective actions taken.

CONCLUSION

The nipple and areola are central players in breastfeeding and are uniquely constructed for their function in delivering breastmilk to an infant. Close attention to the care of the nipple and areola are important to assure that a mother does not wean prematurely due to pain or conditions of the nipple/areolar complex that are left unremedied. Effective support from the clinician often spells the difference between untimely weaning and a long happy breastfeeding experience.

ADDITIONAL RESOURCES

West, D., & Marasco, L. (2008). *The breastfeeding mother's guide to making more milk.* New York: McGraw-Hill.

West, D. (2001). *Defining your own success: Breastfeeding after breast reduction surgery.* Schaumburg, IL: La Leche League International.

West, D., & Hirsch, E.M. (2008). *Breastfeeding after breast and nipple procedures.* Amarillo, TX: Hale Publishing.

Breastfeeding After Breast Reduction Website

www.bfar.org

Low Milk Supply Website

www.lowmilksupply.org

Mothers Overcoming Breastfeeding Issues Website

www.mobimotherhood.org

REFERENCES

Abou-Dakn, M., Schafer-Graf, U., & Wockel, A. (2009). Psychological stress and breast diseases during lactation. *Breastfeeding Review, 17,* 19-26.

Abramson, D.J. (1975). Bilateral intra-areolar polythelia. *Archives of Surgery, 110,* 1255.

Adam, B., Baillie, G.S., & Douglas, L.J. (2002). Mixed species biofilms of Candida albicans and Staphylococcus epidermidis. *Journal of Medical Microbiology, 51,* 344-349.

Ahluwalia, I.B., Morrow, B., & Hsia, J. (2005). Why do women stop breastfeeding? Findings from the pregnancy risk assessment and monitoring system. *Pediatrics, 116,* 1408-1412.

Ahmed, O.A., & Kolhe, P.S. (2000). Comparison of nipple and areolar sensation after breast reduction by free nipple graft and inferior pedicle techniques. *British Journal of Plastic Surgery, 53,* 126–129.

Ahurjai, T., & Natsheh, F.M. (2003). Plants used in cosmetics. *Phytotherapy Research, 17,* 987-1000.

Akkuzu, G., & Taskin, L. (2000). Impacts of breast-care techniques on prevention of possible postpartum nipple problems. *Professional Care of Mother and Child, 10,* 38-41.

Alexander, A., Dowling, D., & Furman, L. (2010). What do pregnant low-income women say about breastfeeding? *Breastfeeding Medicine, 5,* 17-23.

Alexander, J., Grant, A., & Campbell. M,J. (1992). Randomized controlled trial of breast shells and Hoffman's exercises for inverted and non-protractile nipples. *British Medical Journal, 304,* 1030–1032.

Al-Qattan, M.M., & Robertson, G.A. (1990). Bilateral chronic infection of the lactosebaceous glands of Montgomery. *Annals of Plastic Surgery, 25,* 491–493.

Al-Waili, N.S. (2005). Mixture of honey, beeswax and olive oil inhibits growth of *Staphylococcus aureus* and *Candida albicans. Archives of Medical Research, 36,* 10-13.

American Academy of Pediatrics. (2001). The transfer of drugs and other chemicals into human milk. *Pediatrics, 108,* 776–789.

American Academy of Pediatrics, Section on Breastfeeding. (2005). Breastfeeding and the use of human milk. *Pediatrics, 115,* 496-506.

Amir, L.H. (1991). Candida and the lactating breast: Predisposing factors. *Journal of Human Lactation, 7,* 177–181.

Amir, L. (1993). Eczema of the nipple and breast: A case report. *Journal of Human Lactation, 9,* 173–175.

Amir, L.H. (2003). Breast pain in lactating women: Mastitis or something else? *Australian Family Physician, 32,* 392–397.

Amir, L. (2004). Nipple pain in breastfeeding. *Australian Family Physician, 33,* 44-45.

Amir, L.H., Dennerstein, L., Garland, S.M., Fisher, J, & Farish, S.J. (1997). Psychological aspects of nipple pain in lactating women. *Breastfeeding Review, 5,* 29–32.

Amir, L.H., Garland, S., Dennerstein, L., & Farish, S. (1996). Candida albicans: Is it associated with nipple pain in lactating women? *Gynecologic and Obstetric Investigation, 41,* 30–34.

Amir, L.H., Garland, S.M., & Lumley, J. (2006). A case-control study of mastitis: nasal carriage of *Staphylococcus aureus. BMC Family Practice, 7,* 57.

Amir, L., & Hoover, K. (2003). *Candidiasis and breastfeeding.* Lactation Consultant Series 2. Schaumburg, IL: La Leche League International.

Amir, L.H., & Pakula, S. (1991). Nipple pain, mastalgia and candidiasis in the lactating breast. *Australian and New Zealand Obstetrics and Gynaecology, 31,* 378–380.

Anderson, J.E., Held, N., & Wright, K. (2004). Raynaud's phenomenon of the nipple: A treatable cause of painful breastfeeding. *Pediatrics, 113,* e360–e364.

Andersson, Y., Lindquist, S., Lagerqvust, C., & Hernell, O. (2000). Lactoferrin is responsible for fungistatic effect of human milk. *Early Human Development, 59,* 95–105.

Andrews, J.I., Fleener, D.K., Messer, S.A., Hansen, W.F., Pfaller, M.A., Diekema, D.J. (2007) The yeast connection: is Candida linked to breastfeeding associated pain? *American Journal of Obstetrics and Gynecology, 197,* 424.e1-4.

Ansara, D., Cohen, M.M., Gallop, R., Kung, R., & Schei, B. (2005). Predictors of women's physical health problems after childbirth. *Journal of Psychosomatic Obstetrics & Gynecology, 26,* 115-125.

Applebaum, R.M. (1969). *Abreast of the times.* Miami, FL: RM Applebaum.

Ardran, G.M., & Kemp, F.H. (1958). A cineradiographic study of breast feeding. *British Journal of Radiology, 31,* 156-162.

Armstrong, M.L., Caliendo, C., & Roberts, A.E. (2006). Pregnancy, lactation and nipple piercings. *AWHONN Lifelines, 10,* 212-217.

Atkinson, L.D. (1979). Prenatal nipple conditioning for breastfeeding. *Nursing Research, 28,* 267-271.

Ballard, J.L., Auer, C.E., & Khoury, J.C. (2002). Ankyloglossia: Assessment, incidence, and the effect of frenuloplasty on the breastfeeding dyad. *Pediatrics, 110*(5) Downloaded from www.pediatrics.org/cgi/contant/full/110/5/e63 on December 13, 2009.

Ballesio, L., Maggi, C., Savelli, S., Angeletti, M., Rabuffi, P., Manganaro, L., et al. (2007). Adjunctive diagnostic value of ultrasonography evaluation in patients with suspected ductal breast disease. *Radiologic Medicine, 112,* 354–365.

Barankin, B., & Gross, M.S. (2004). Nipple and areolar eczema in the breastfeeding woman. *Journal of Cutaneous Medicine and Surgery, 8,* 126–130.

Baratelli, G.M., & Vischi, S. (1999). Unilateral intra-areolar polythelia: A rare anomaly. *The Breast, 8,* 51-52.

Baumann, L.S. (2007). Less known botanical cosmeceuticals. *Dermatological Therapy, 39,* 330-342.

Benbow, M., & Vardy-White, C. (2004). Study into the effectiveness of Mothermates. *British Journal of Midwifery, 12,* 244-248.

Blair, A., Cadwell, K., Turner-Maffei, C., & Brimdyr, K. (2003). The relationship between positioning, the breastfeeding dynamic, the latching process and pain in breastfeeding mothers with sore nipples. *Breastfeeding Review, 11,* 5–10.

Bland, K.I., & Romnell, L.J. (1991). Congenital and acquired disturbances of breast development and growth. In K.I. Bland & E.M. Copeland III (Eds.), *The breast: Comprehensive management of benign and malignant diseases.* Philadelphia: Saunders.

Blech, H., Friebe, K., & Krause, W. (2004). Inflammation of Montgomery glands. Acta *Dermato Venereologica, 84,* 93-94.

Blumenthal, M., Goldberg, A., & Brinckmann, J. (2000). *Herbal medicine: expanded Commission E Monographs.* Newton, MA. Integrative Medicine Communications, 297-303.

Bodley, V., & Powers, D. (1996). Long-term nipple shield use—a positive perspective. *Journal of Human Lactation, 12,* 301–304.

Bodley, V., & Powers, D. (1997). Long-term treatment of a breastfeeding mother with fluconazole-resolved nipple pain caused by yeast: A case study. *Journal of Human Lactation, 13,* 307–311.

Bracket, V.H. (1988). Eczema of the nipple/areola area. *Journal of Human Lactation, 4,* 167–169.

Brent, N.B. (2001). Thrush in the breastfeeding dyad: Results of a survey on diagnosis and treatment. *Clinical Pediatrics, 40,* 503–506.

Brent, N., Rudy, S.J., Redd, B., Rudy, T.E., & Roth, L.A. (1998). Sore nipples in breastfeeding women: A clinical trial of wound dressings vs conventional care. *Archives of Pediatric and Adolescent Medicine, 152,* 1077–1082.

Brigham, M. (1996). Mothers' reports of the outcome of nipple shield use. *Journal of Human Lactation, 12,* 291–297.

Briggs, J. (2003). The management of nipple pain and/or trauma associated with breastfeeding. *Best Practice, 7,* 1–6.

Brook, I., & Gober, A.E. (1997). Bacterial colonization of pacifiers of infants with acute otitis media. *Journal of Laryngology and Otology, 111*, 614–615.

Brown, J., & Schwartz, R.A. (2003). Supernumerary nipples: An overview. *Cutis, 71*,344-346.

Brown, M.S., & Hurlock, J.T. (1975). Preparation of the breast for breastfeeding. *Nursing Research, 24,* 448-451.

Brzozowski, D., Niessen, M., Evans, H.B., & Hurst, L.N. (2000). Breastfeeding after inferior pedicle reduction mammaplasty. *Plastic Reconstructive Surgery, 105*, 530–534.

Buchko, B.L., Pugh, L.C., Bishop, B.A., Cochran, J.F., Smith, L.R., & Lerew, D.J. (1994). Comfort measures in breastfeeding, primiparous women. *Journal of Obstetric, Gynecologic and Neonatal Nursing, 23*, 46-52.

Cable, B., Stewart, M., & Davis, J. (1997). Nipple wound care: A new approach to an old problem. *Journal of Human Lactation, 13*, 313–318.

Cadwell, K. (1981). Improving nipple graspability for success at breastfeeding. *Journal of Obstetric Gynecologic and Neonatal Nursing, 10*, 277–279.

Cadwell, K., Turner-Maffei, C., Blair, A., Brimdyr, K., & McInerney, Z. (2004). Pain reduction and treatment of sore nipples in nursing mothers. *Journal of Perinatal Education, 13*, 29-35.

Casey, H.D., Chasan, P.E., & Chick, L.R. (1996). Familial polythelia without associated anomalies. *Annals of Plastic Surgery, 36*, 101-104.

Carmichael, A.R., & Dixon, J.M. (2002). Is lactation mastitis and shooting breast pain experienced by women during lactation caused by Candida albicans? *Breast, 11,* 88-90.

Cellini, A., & Offidani, A. (1988). Familial supernumerary nipples. *American Journal of Medical Genetics, 31*, 631-635.

Cherchel, A., Azzam, C., & De May, A. (2007). Breastfeeding after vertical reduction mammaplasty using a superior pedicle. *Journal of Plastic Reconstructive Aesthetic Surgery, 60*, 465-470.

Chertok, I.R., Schneider, J., & Blackburn, S. (2006). A pilot study of maternal and term infant outcomes associated with ultrathin nipple shield use. *Journal of Obstetric Gynecologic and Neonatal Nursing, 35*, 265–272.

Chetwynd, E.M., Ives, T.J., Payne, P.M., & Edens-Bartholomew, N. (2002). Fluconazole for postpartum candidal mastitis and infant thrush. *Journal of Human Lactation, 18*, 168–171.

Chiummariello, S., Cigna, E., Buccheri, E.M., Dessy, L.A., Alfano, C., & Scuderi, N. (2008). Breastfeeding after reduction mammaplasty using different techniques. *Aesthetic Plastic Surgery, 32*, 294-297.

Coates, M-M. (1992). Nipple pain related to vasospasm in the nipple? *Journal of Human Lactation, 8*, 153.

Coca, K.P., & Abrao, A.C.F.V. (2008). An evaluation of the effect of lanolin in healing nipple injuries. *Acta Paul Enferm, 21*, 11-16.

Coca, K.P., Gamba, M.A., de Souza e Silva, R., & Abrao, A.C.F.V. (2009). Factors associated with nipple trauma in the maternity unit. *Journal of Pediatrics (Rio J), 85*, 341-345.

Colson, S.D., Meek, J.H., & Hawdon, J.M. (2008). Optimal positions for the release of primitive neonatal reflexes stimulating breastfeeding. *Early Human Development, 84*, 441-449.

Colmina, E., Marion, K., Renaud, F.N.R., Dore, J., Bergeron, E., & Freney, J. (2006). Pacifiers: A microbial reservoir. *Nursing and Health Sciences, 8,* 216-223.

Cooper A.P. (1840). *Anatomy of the breast.* London: Longman, Orme, Green, Browne and Longmans.

Cooper, W.O., Atherton, H.D., Kahana, M., & Kotagal, U.R. (1995). Increased incidence of severe breastfeeding malnutrition and hypernatremia in a metropolitan area. *Pediatrics, 96*, 957–960.

Cotch, M.F., Hillier, S.L., Gibbs, R.S., & Eschenbach, D.A. (1998). Epidemiology and outcomes associated with moderate to heavy Candida colonization during pregnancy. *American Journal of Obstetrics and Gynecology, 178*, 374–380.

Cotterman, K.J. (2003). Too swollen to latch on? Try reverse pressure softening first. *Leaven, April/May*, 38–40.

Cotterman, K.J. (2004). Reverse pressure softening: A simple tool to prepare areola for easier latching during engorgement. *Journal of Human Lactation, 20*, 227-237.

Cricco-Lizza, R. (2004). Infant feeding beliefs and experiences of black women enrolled in WIC in the New York metropolitan area. *Quality Health Research, 14,* 1197-1210.

Cruz, N.I., & Korchin, L. (2007). Lactational performance after breast reduction with different pedicles. *Plastic Reconstructive Surgery, 120*, 35-40.

Darwazeh, AM., & al-Bashir, A. (1995). Oral candidal flora in healthy infants. *Journal Oral Pathology Medicine, 24*, 361–364.

da Silveira, L.C., Charone, S., Maia, L.C., Soares, R.M., & Portela, M.B. (2009). Biofilm formation by Candida species on silicone surfaces and latex pacifier nipples: An in vitro study. *Journal of Clinical Pediatric Dentistry, 33*, 235-240.

Dean, N., Haynes, J., Brennan, J., Neild, T., Goddard, C., Dearman, B., et al. (2005). Nipple-areolar pigmentation: Histology and potential for reconstitution in breast reconstruction. *British Journal of Plastic Surgery, 58*, 202-208.

Dekio, S., Kawasaki, Y., & Jidoi, J. (1986). Herpes simplex on nipples inoculated from herpes gingivostomatitis of a baby. *Clinical and Experimental Dermatology,*

11, 664–666.

Dewey, K.G., Nommsen-Rivers. L., Heinig, M.J., & Cohen R.J. (2003). Risk factors for suboptimal infant breastfeeding behavior, delayed onset of lactation, and excess neonatal weight loss. *Pediatrics, 112*, 607–619.

Dinsmoor, M.J., Viloria, R., Lief, L., & Elder, S. (2005). Use of intrapartum antibiotics and the incidence of postnatal maternal and neonatal yeast infections. *Obstetrics and Gynecology, 106*, 19-22.

Dodd, V., & Chalmers, C. (2003). Comparing the use of hydrogel dressings to lanolin ointment with lactating mothers. *Journal of Obstetric, Gynecologic, and Neonatal Nursing, 32*, 486-494.

Dollberg, S., Botzer, E., Grunis, E., & Mimouni, F.B. (2006). Immediate nipple pain relief after frenotomy in breastfed infants with ankyloglossia: A randomized, prospective study. *Journal of Pediatric Surgery, 41*, 1598-1600.

Doucet, S., Soussignan, R., Sagot, P. & Schaal, B. (2007). The "smellscape" of mother's breast: Effects of odor masking and selective unmasking on neonatal arousal, oral, and visual responses. *Developmental Psychobiology, 49*, 129-138.

Doucet, S., Soussignan, R., Sagot, P., & Schaal, B. (2009). The secretion of areolar (Montgomery's) glands from lactating women elicits selective, unconditional responses in neonates. *PLoS ONE, 4*(10), e7579. Retrieved October 25, 2009 from http://www.plosone.org/article/info:doi%2F10.1371%2Fjournal.pone.0007579.

Drewett, R., Kahn, H., Parkhurst, S., & Whiteley, S. (1987). Pain during breastfeeding: The first three months. *Journal of Reproductive Infant Psychology, 5*, 183–186.

Eastwood, J., Offutt, C., Menon, K., Keel, M., Hrncirova, P., Novotny, M.V., et al. (2007). Identification of markers for nipple epidermis: Changes in expression during pregnancy and lactation. *Differentiation, 75*, 75-83.

Eglash, A., Plane, M.B., & Mundt, M. (2006). History, physical and laboratory findings, and clinical outcomes of lactating women treated with antibiotics for chronic breast and/or nipple pain. *Journal of Human Lactation, 22*, 429-433.

Eglash, A., & Proctor, R. (2007). A breastfeeding mother with chronic breast pain. *Breastfeeding Medicine, 2*, 99-103.

Ehrenkranz, R., Ackerman, B., & Hulse, J. (1989). Nifedipine transfer into human milk. *Journal of Pediatrics, 114*, 478–480.

Ellepola, A.N., Panagoda, G.J., & Samaranayake, L.P. (1999). Adhesion of oral Candida species to human buccal epithelial cells following brief exposure to nystatin. *Oral Microbiology Immunology, 14*, 358–363.

Emslie, M. (1931). *Breast feeding.* Oxford University Press.

Epstein, A.N., Blass, E.M., Batshaw, M.L., & Parks, A.D. (1970). The vital role of saliva as a mechanical sealant for suckling in the rat. *Physiology and Behavior,*

5, 1395-1398.

Eriksson, M., Lindh, B., Uvnas-Moberg, K., & Hokfelt, T. (1996). Distribution and origin of peptide-containing nerve fibers in the rat and human mammary gland. *Neuroscience, 70*, 227-245.

Evans, P.R., & Mackeith, R. (1954). *Infant feeding and feeding difficulties*. J. & A. Churchill, Ltd.

Falkenberry, S.S. (2002). Nipple discharge. *Obstetrics and Gynecology Clinics of North America, 29*, 21-29.

Ferrara, P., Giorgio, V., Vitelli, O., Gatto, A., Romano, V., Bufalo, F.D., et al. (2009). Polythelia: Still a marker of urinary tract anomalies in children? *Scandinavian Journal of Urology and Nephrology, 43,* 47-50.

Fetherston, C. (1998). Risk factors for lactation mastitis. *Journal of Human Lactation, 14*, 101–109.

Fildes, V. (1986). *Breasts, bottles and babies: A history of infant feeding*. Edinburgh: Edinburgh University press.

Fleming, P.A. (1984). Brief reports: The effect of prenatal nipple conditioning on postpartum nipple pain of breastfeeding women. *Health Care for Women International, 5*, 453-457.

Foxman, B., D'Arcy, H., Gillespie, B., Bobo, J., & Schwartz, K. (2002). Lactation mastitis: Occurrence and medical management among 946 breastfeeding women in the United States. *American Journal of Epidemiology, 155*, 115-116.

Gangal, H.T., & Gangal, M.H. (1978). Suction method for correcting flat nipples or inverted nipples. *Plastic and Reconstructive Surgery, 61*, 294–296.

Gans, B. (1958). Breast and nipple pain in early stages of lactation. *British Medical Journal, 2*(5100), 830-832.

Garbin, C.P., Deacon, J.P., Rowan, M.K., Hartmann, P.E., & Geddes, D.T. (2009). Association of nipple piercing with abnormal milk production and breastfeeding. *Journal of the American Medical Association, 301*, 2550-2551.

Garrison, C.P. (2002). Nipple vasospasms, Raynaud's syndrome, and nifedipine. *Journal of Human Lactation, 18,* 382-385.

Geddes, D.T., Kent, J.C., Mitoulas, L.R., & Hartmann, P.E. (2008a). Tongue movement and intra-oral vacuum in breastfeeding infants. *Early Human Development, 84*, 471-477.

Geddes, D.T., Langton, D.B., Gollow, I., Jacobs, L.A., Hartmann, P.E., & Simmer, K. (2008b). Frenulotomy for breastfeeding infants with ankyloglossia: Effect on milk removal and sucking mechanism as imaged by ultrasound. *Pediatrics, 122,* e188-e194.

Going, J.J., & Moffat, D.F. (2004). Escaping from flatland: Clinical and biological aspects of human mammary duct anatomy in three dimensions. *Journal of*

Pathology, 203, 538–544.

Going, J.J., & Mohun, T.J. (2006). Human breast duct anatomy, the 'sick' lobe hypothesis and intraductal approaches to breast cancer. *Breast Cancer Research and Treatment, 97*, 285-291.

Gonzalez, F., Brown, F.E., Gold, M.E., Walton, R.L., & Shafer, B. (1993). Preoperative and postoperative nipple-areola sensibility in patients undergoing reduction mammaplasty. *Plastic Reconstructive Surgery, 92*, 809–814.

Gooding, M.J., Finlay, J., Shipley, J.A., Halliwell, M., & Duck, F.A. (2010). Three-dimensional ultrasound imaging of mammary ducts in lactating women. *Journal of Ultrasound medicine, 29*, 95-103.

Graves, S., Wright, W., Harman, R., & Bailey, S. (2003). Painful nipples in nursing mothers: Fungal or staphylococcal? *Australian Family Physician, 32*, 570–571.

Griffiths, D.M. (2004). Do tongue ties affect breastfeeding? *Journal of Human Lactation, 20*, 409-414.

Grimes, D.A., & Schulz, K.F. (2002). Uses and abuses of screening tests. *Lancet, 359*, 881–884.

Gunther, M. (1945). Sore nipples: Causes and prevention. *Lancet, ii*, 590–593.

Gunther, M. (1970). *Infant feeding.* London, UK: Metheun.

Hale, T.W. (2008). *Medications and mother's milk.* 13th ed. Amarillo, TX: Hale Publishing.

Hale, T.W., Bateman, T.L., Finkelman, M.A., & Berens, P.D. (2009). The absence of *Candida albicans* in milk samples of women with clinical symptoms of ductal candidiasis. *Breastfeeding Medicine, 4*, 57-61.

Hale, T.W., & Berens, P. (2002). *Clinical therapy in breastfeeding patients. 2nd ed.* Amarillo, TX: Pharmasoft Publishing.

Hallock, G.G. (1992). Prediction of nipple viability following reduction mammoplasty using laser Doppler flowmetry. *Annals of Plastic Surgery, 29*, 457–460.

Han, S., & Hong, Y. (1999). The inverted nipple: Its grading and surgical correction. *Plastic Reconstructive Surgery, 104*, 389-395.

Heads, J., & Higgins, L.C. (1995). Perceptions and correlates of nipple pain. *Breastfeeding Review, 3*, 59–64.

Henderson, A., Stamp, G., & Pincombe, J. (2001). Postpartum positioning and attachment education for increasing breastfeeding: A randomized trial. *Birth, 28*, 236-242.

Hewat, R.J., & Ellis, D.J. (1987). A comparison of the effectiveness of two methods of nipple care. *Birth, 14*, 41-45.

Hill, P.D., & Humenick, S.S. (1993). Nipple pain during breastfeeding: The first two weeks and beyond. *Journal of Perinatal Education, 2*, 21–35.

Hoffman, J.B. (1953). A suggested treatment for inverted nipples. *American Journal of Obstetrics and Gynecology, 66*, 346-348.

Hogan, M., Westcott, C., & Griffiths, M. (2005). Randomised controlled division of tongue tie in infants with breastfeeding problems. *Journal of Paediatric and Child Health, 41*, 246-250.

Hoppe, J.E. (1997). Treatment of oropharyngeal candidiasis in immunocompetent infants: A randomized multicenter study of miconazol gel vs. nystatin suspension. *Pediatric Infectious Disease Journal, 16*, 288-293.

Hoppe, J.E., & Hahn, H. (1996). Randomized comparison of two nystatin oral gels with miconazole oral gel for treatment of oral thrush in infants. *Infection, 24*, 136–139.

Hsu, S. (2005). Green tea and the skin. *Journal of the American Academy of Dermatology*, 52, 1049-1059.

Hsu, S., Bollag, W.B., Lewis, J., Huang, Q., Singh, B., Sharawy, M., et al. (2003). Green tea polyphenols induce differentiation and proliferation in epidermal keratinocytes. *Journal of Pharmacology and Experimental Therapeutics, 306*, 29-34.

Huang Z-R., Lin, Y-K, & Fang, J-Y. (2009). Biological and pharmacological activities of squalene and related compounds: Potential uses in cosmetic dermatology. *Molecules, 14*, 540-554.

Huggins, K.E., & Billon, S.F. (1993). Twenty cases of persistent sore nipples: Collaboration between lactation consultant and dermatologist. *Journal of Human Lactation, 9*, 155-160.

Humenick, S., & van Steenkiste, S. (1983). Early indicators of breastfeeding progress. *Issues in Comprehensive Pediatric Nursing, 6*, 205–215.

Hurley, K.M., Black, M.M., Papas, M.A., Quigg, A.M. (2008). Variation on breastfeeding behaviours, perceptions, and experiences by race/ethnicity among a low-income statewide sample of Special Supplemental Nutrition program for Women, Infants, and Children (WIC) participants in the United States. *Maternal Child Nutrition, 4*, 95-105.

Hurst, N.M. (1996). Lactation after augmentation mammoplasty. *Obstetrics and Gynecology, 87*, 30-34.

Hussain, A.N., Policarpio, C., & Vincent, M.T. (2006). Evaluating nipple discharge. *Obstetrics and Gynecology Survey, 61*, 278-83.

Hytten, F.E., & Baird, D. (1958). The development of the nipple in pregnancy. *Lancet, 1(7032)*, 1201-1204.

Inch, S. (1989). Antenatal preparation for breastfeeding. In I. Chalmers, M. Enkin, & M.J.N.C. Keirse (Eds.), *Effective care in pregnancy and childbirth.* Oxford: Oxford University Press.

Islam, Q.T., Karimeddini, M.K., Spencer, R.P., Kurtzman, S.H., & Vento, J.A. (2000). Positive Tc-99m MIBI breast study related to a psoriatic lesion. *Clinical Nuclear Medicine, 25,* 374.

Jaber, L., & Merlob, P. (1988). The prevalence of supernumerary nipples in Arab infants and children. *European Journal of Pediatrics, 147,* 443.

Jacobs, L.A., Dickinson, J.E., Hart, P.D., Doherty, D.A., & Faulkner, S.J. (2007). Normal nipple position in term infants measured on breastfeeding ultrasound. *Journal of Human Lactation, 23,* 52-59.

Jacobs, V.R., Golombeck, K., Jonat, W., & Kiechle, M. (2003). Mastitis nonpuerperalis after nipple piercing: Time to act. *International Journal of Fertility and Women's Medicine, 48,* 226–231.

Jamali, F., Ricci, A., & Deckers, P. (1996). Paget's disease of the nipple-areola complex. *Surgery Clinics of North America, 76,* 365–381.

Jevitt, C., Hernandez, I., & Groer, M. (2007). Lactation complicated by overweight and obesity: Supporting the mother and newborn. *Journal of Midwifery & Women's Health,* 52, 606-613.

Johnson, C.A., Felson, B., & Jolles, H. (1986). Polythelia (supernumerary nipple): An update. *Southern Medical Journal, 79,* 1106-1110.

Johnstone, H.A., & Marcinak, J.F. (1990). Candidiasis in the breastfeeding mother and infant. *Journal of Obstetric, Gynecologic, and Neonatal Nursing, 19,* 171–173.

Jones, E., Dimmock, P.W., & Spencer, S.A. (2001). A randomised controlled trial to compare methods of milk expression after preterm delivery. *Archives of Disease in Children. Fetal Neonatal Edition, 85,* F91–F95.

Jones, E., & Hilton, S. (2009). Correctly fitting breast shields are the key to lactation success for pump dependent mothers following preterm delivery. *Journal of Neonatal Nursing, 15,* 14-17.

Jones, L. (1999). Pierced nipples and breastfeeding: Achieving compromise. *Practicing Midwife, 2,* 16-17.

Kajava, Y. (1915). The proportions of supernumerary nipples in the Finnish population. *Duodecim, 31,* 143-170.

Kenney, R.D., Flippo, J.L., & Black, E.B. (1987). Supernumerary nipples and renal anomalies in neonates. *American Journal of Diseases in Children, 141,* 987-988.

Kesaree, N. (1993). Treatment of inverted nipples using disposable syringe. *Indian Pediatrics, 30,* 429-430.

Kesaree, N., Banapurmath, C.R., Banapurmath, S., & Shamanur, K. (1993). Treatment of inverted nipples using a disposable syringe. *Journal of Human Lactation, 9,* 27–29.

Khoo, A.K., Dabbas, N., Sudhakaran, N., Ade-Ajayi, N., & Patel, S. (2009). Nipple pain at presentation predicts success of tongue-tie division for breastfeeding problems. *European Journal of Pediatric Surgery, 19,* 370-373.

Kim H.S., Noh, S.U., Han Y.W., Kim, K.M., Kang, H., Kim, H.O., et al. (2009). Therapeutic effects of topical application of ozone on acute cutaneous wound healing. *Journal of Korean Medical Science, 24,* 368-374.

Kinlay, J.R., O'Connell, D.L., & Kinlay, S. (2001). Risk factors for mastitis in breastfeeding women: Results of a prospective cohort study. *Australia/New Zealand Journal of Public Health, 25,* 115–120.

Kline, T.S., & Lash, S.R. (1962). Nipple secretion in pregnancy: A cytologic and histologic study. *American Journal of Clinical Pathology, 37,* 626.

Lafreniere, R. (1990). Bloody nipple discharge during pregnancy: A rationale for conservative treatment. *Journal of Surgical Oncology, 43,* 228.

Lavergne, N.A. (1997). Does application of tea bags to sore nipples while breastfeeding provide effective relief? *Journal of Obstetric, Gynecologic, and Neonatal Nursing, 26,* 53-58.

Lawlor-Smith, L., & Lawlor-Smith, C. (1996). Nipple vasospasm in the breastfeeding woman. *Breastfeeding Review, 4,* 37–39.

Lawlor-Smith, L., & Lawlor-Smith, C. (1997). Vasospasm of the nipple—A manifestation of Raynaud's phenomenon: Case reports. *British Medical Journal, 314,* 844–845.

Lawrence, R.A, & Lawrence, R.M. (2005). *Breastfeeding: A guide for the medical profession.* 6th ed. Philadelphia, PA: Elsevier Mosby.

L'Esperance, C. (1980). Pain or pleasure: The dilemma of early breastfeeding. *Birth, 7,* 21–26.

Lever, R., Hadley, K., Downey, D., & Mackie, R. (1988). Staphylococcal colonization in atopic dermatitis and the effect of topical mupirocin therapy. *British Journal of Dermatology, 119,* 189–198.

Li, X., Zhang, H., Li, R., et al. (2000). Experience in treating 260 cases of fissure of nipple with MEBO. *The Chinese Journal of Burns, Wounds & Surface Ulcers, 12,* 32-33.

Livingstone, V., & Stringer, L.J. (1999). The treatment of Staphylococcus aureus infected sore nipples: A randomized comparative study. *Journal of Human Lactation, 15,* 241–246.

Livingstone, V.H., Willis, C.E., & Berkowitz, J. (1996). Staphylococcus aureus and sore nipples. *Canadian Family Physician, 42,* 654–659.

Lochner, J.E., Livingston, C.J., & Judkins, D.Z. (2009). Which interventions are best for alleviating nipple pain in nursing mothers? *Journal of Family Practice, 58*(11), retrieved from http://www.jfponline.com/Pages.asp?AID=8105 on December 31, 2009.

Lopez, J.L.A., Garcia, L., Elena, E., Benito, P., & Juan A.D. (2006). Unilateral dichotomy of nipple (intraareolar polythelia) and areola: Report of a case and surgical correction. *Aesthetic Plastic Surgery, 30*, 494-496.

Lopez, J.L.A., Sorando, E.E., Martinez, L.G., & Bravo, T.R. (2005). Intra-areolar polythelia with a partly doubled areola without any other malformations. *Dermatology, 211*, 383-384.

Love, S.M., & Barsky, S.H. (2004). Anatomy of the nipple and breast ducts revisited. *Cancer, 101*,1947–1957.

Macfarlane, A.J. (1975). Olfaction in the development of social preferences in human neonate. In Elsevier (Ed.), *Parent-infant interaction* (pp.103-117). Amsterdam: Ciba Foundation Symposia.

MAIN Trial Collaborative Group. (1994). Preparing for breastfeeding: Treatment of inverted and non-protractile nipples in pregnancy. *Midwifery, 10*, 200-214.

Makin, J.W., & Porter, R.H. (1989). Attractiveness of lactating females' breast odors to neonates. *Child Development, 60*, 803-810.

Manizheh, S.M., Mohammad, R.R., Abbas D., et al. (2007a). Effect of peppermint water on prevention of nipple cracks in lactating primiparous women: a randomized controlled trial. *International Breastfeeding Journal, 2*, 7.

Manizheh, S.M., Mohammad, R.R., Ali, N., et al. (2007b). A randomized trial of peppermint gel, lanolin ointment, and placebo gel to prevent nipple crack in primiparous breastfeeding women. *Medical Science Monitor, 13*, CR406-CR411.

Manning, D.J., Coughlin, R.P., & Poskitt, E.M.E. (1985). Candida in mouth or on dummy? *Archives of Disease in Children, 60*, 381–382.

Martin, J. (2004). Is nipple piercing compatible with breastfeeding? *Journal of Human Lactation, 20*, 319–321.

Mathes, S.J., Seyfer, A.E., & Miranda, E.P. (2006). Congenital anomalies of the chest wall. In S.J. Mathes & V.R. Hentz (Eds.), *Plastic surgery VI*. Philadelphia: Elsevier, pp. 457–537.

Mattos-Graner, R.O., de Moraes, A.B., Rontani, R.M., & Birman, E.G. (2001). Relation of oral yeast infection in Brazilian infants and the use of a pacifier. *ASDC Journal of Dentistry for Children, 68*, 33–36.

McClellan, H.L., Geddes, D.T., Kent, J.C., Garbin, C.P., Mitoulas, L.R., & Hartmann, P.E. (2008). Infants of mothers with persistent nipple pain exert strong sucking vacuums. *Acta Paediatrica, 97*, 1205-1209.

McGeorge, D.D. (1994). The "niplette": An instrument for the non-surgical correction of inverted nipples. *British Journal of Plastic Surgery 47*, 46–49.

McGovern, P., Dowd, B., Gjerdingen, D., Gross, C.R., Kenney, S., Ukestad, L., McCaffrey, D., et al. (2006). Postpartum health of employed mothers 5 weeks after childbirth. *Annals of Family Medicine, 4*, 159-167.

Meier, P., Motyhowski, J., & Zuleger, J. (2004). Choosing a correctly fitted breast shield for milk expression. *Medela Messenger, 21*, 8-9.

Melli, M.S., Mohammad, R.R., Abbas D., Madarek, E., Kargar Maher, M.H., Ghasemzadeh, A., et al. (2007a). Effect of peppermint water on prevention of nipple cracks in lactating primiparous women: A randomized controlled trial. *International Breastfeeding Journal, 2*, 7.

Melli, M.S., Rashidi, M.R., Nokhoodchi, A., Tagavi, S., Farzadi, L., Sadaghat, K., et al. (2007b). A randomized trial of peppermint gel, lanolin ointment, and placebo gel to prevent nipple crack in primiparous breastfeeding women. *Medical Science Monitor, 13*, CR406-CR411.

Messner, A.H., Lalakea, M.H., Aby, J., MacMahon, J., & Blair, E. (2000). Ankyloglossia incidence and associated feeding difficulties. *Archives of Otolaryngology Head Neck Surgery, 126*, 36-39.

Miller, V., & Riordan, J. (2004). Treating postpartum breast edema with areolar compression. *Journal of Human Lactation, 20*, 223-226.

Mimica-Dukic, N., & Bozin, B. (2008). Mentha L. species (Lamiaceae) as promising sources of bioactive secondary metabolites. *Current Pharmaceutical Design, 14*, 3141-3150.

Mimica-Dukić N., Bozin, B., Soković, M., Mihajlović, B., & Matavulj. M. (2003). Antimicrobial and antioxidant activities of three Mentha species essential oils. *Planta Medica, 69*, 413-419.

Mimouni, F., Merlob, P., & Reisner, S.H. (1983). Occurrence of supernumerary nipples in newborns. *American Journal of Diseases in Children, 137*, 952-953.

Mitz, V., & Lalardie, J.P. (1977). A propos de la vascularisation et de l'innervation sensitive du sein. *Senologia, 2*, 33-39.

Moffat, D.F., & Going, J.J. (1996). Three dimensional anatomy of complete duct systems in human breast: Pathological and developmental implications. *Journal of Clinical Pathology, 49*, 48-52.

Mofid, M.M., Klatsky, S.A., Singh, N.K., & Nahabedian, M.Y. (2006). Nipple-areola complex sensitivity after primary breast augmentation: A comparison of periareolar and inframammary incision approaches. *Plastic Reconstructive Surgery, 117*, 1694-1698.

Mohammadzadeh, A., Farhat, A., & Esmaeily, H. (2005). The effect of breast milk and lanolin on sore nipples. *Saudi Medical Journal, 26*, 1231-1234.

Mohrbacher, Nancy. (2010) *Breastfeeding answers made simple: A guide for helping mothers.* Amarillo,TX: Hale Publishing.

Monroe, D. (2007). Looking for chinks in the armor of bacterial biofilms. *PLoS Biology, 5*, e307 doi:10.1371/journal.pbio.0050307.

Montagna, W. (1970). Histology and cytochemistry of human skin XXXV. The nipple and areola. *British Journal of Dermatology, 83*, 2-13.

Montagna, W., & MacPherson, E.E. (1974). Some neglected aspects of the human breasts. *Journal of Investigative Dermatology, 63*, 10-16.

Montagna, W., & Yun, J.S. (1972). The glands of Montgomery. *British Journal of Dermatology, 86*, 126-133.

Morino, C., & Winn, S.M. (2007). Raynaud's phenomenon of the nipples: An elusive diagnosis. *Journal of Human Lactation, 23*, 191-193.

Morland-Schultz, K., & Hill, P.D. (2005). Prevention of and therapies for nipple pain: A systematic review. *Journal of Obstetric, Gynecologic, and Neonatal Nursing, 34*, 428-437.

Morrill, J.F., Heinig, M.J., Pappagianis, D., & Dewey, K.G. (2005). Risk factors for mammary candidosis among lactating women. *Journal of Obstetric Gynecologic and Neonatal Nursing, 34,* 37–45.

Morrill, J.F., Heinig, M.J., Pappagianis, D., & Dewey K.G. (2004). Diagnostic value of signs and symptoms of mammary candidosis among lactating women. *Journal of Human Lactation, 20*, 288–295.

Morrill, J.M., Pappagianis, D., Heinig, M.J., Lönnerdal, B., & Dewey, K.G. (2003). Detecting *Candida albicans* in human milk. *Journal of Clinical Microbiology, 41*, 475–478.

Murimi, M., Dodge, C.M., Pope, J., Erickson, D. (2010). Factors that influence breastfeeding decisions among Special Supplemental Nutrition Program for Women, Infants, and Children participants from central Louisiana. *Journal of the American Dietetic Association, 110*, 624-627.

Nahabedian, M.Y., & Mofid, M.M. (2002). Viability and sensation of the nipple-areolar complex after reduction mammaplasty. *Annals of Plastic Surgery, 49*, 24–31.

Neifert, M., & Seacat, J. (1986). Medical management of successful breastfeeding. *Pediatric Clinics of North America, 33*, 743–762.

Newman, J., & Kernerman, E. (2008). Candida protocol. Accessed from http://www.drjacknewman.com/help/Candida-Protocol.asp on January 18, 2010.

Newton, N. (1952). Nipple pain and nipple damage: Problems in management of breastfeeding. *Journal of Pediatrics, 41*, 411-423.

Newton, M., & Newton, N.R. (1948). The let-down reflex in human lactation. *Journal of Pediatrics, 33*, 698.

Nickell, W.B., & Skelton, J. (2005). Breast fat and fallacies: More than 100 years of anatomical fantasy. *Journal of Human Lactation, 21*, **126-130.**

Nishitani, S., Miyamura, T., Tagawa, M., Sumi, M., Takase, R., Doi, H., et al. (2009). The calming effect of a maternal breast milk odor on the human newborn infant. *Neuroscience Research, 63*, 66-71.

Noble, R. (1991). Milk under the skin (milk blister)—a simple problem causing other breast conditions. *Breastfeeding Review, 2,* 118–119.

O'Callaghan, M.A. (1981). Atypical discharge from the breast during pregnancy and/or lactation. *Australian New Zealand Journal of Obstetrics and Gynecology, 21,* 214-216.

Odds, F.C. (1994). Candida species and virulence. *American Society of Microbiology News, 60,* 313–318.

Ohtake, T., Kimijima, I., Fukushima, T., Yasuda, M., Sekikawa, K., Takenoshita, S., et al. (2001). Computer-assisted complete three-dimensional reconstruction of the mammary ductal/lobular systems: Implications of ductal anastomoses for breast-conserving surgery. *Cancer, 91,* 2263–2272.

Olsen, N., & Nielson, S.L. (1978). Prevalence of primary Raynaud's phenomenon in young females. *Scandinavian Journal of Clinical Laboratory Investigation, 37,* 761–776.

Onesti, M.G., Anniboletti, T., Spinelli, G., & Meggiorini, M.L. (2008). Bilateral intra-areolar polythelia: Report of a rare case. *Aesthetic Plastic Surgery,* DOI 10.1007/s00266-008-9277-9. Published online November 27, 2008.

Osterman, K.L., & Rahm, V.A. (2000). Lactation mastitis: Bacterial cultivation of breast milk, symptoms, treatment, and outcome. *Journal of Human Lactation, 16,* 297–302.

Osther, P., Balslev, E., & Blichert-toft, M. (1990). Paget's disease of the nipple: A continuing enigma. *Acta Chirurgica Scandinavica, 156,* 343–352.

Otte, M.J. (1975). Correcting inverted nipples—An aid to breastfeeding. *American Journal of Maternal Child Nursing, 75,* 454–456.

Page, S.M., & McKenna, D.S. (2006). Vasospasm of the nipple presenting as painful lactation. *Obstetrics and Gynecology, 108,* 806-808.

Panjaitan, M., Amir, L.H., Costs, A-M., Rudland, E., & Tabrizi, S. (2008). Polymerase chain reaction in detection of *Candida albicans* for confirmation of clinical diagnosis of nipple thrush. *Breastfeeding Medicine [letter], 3,* 185-187.

Park, H.S., Yoon, C.H., & Kim, H.J. (1999). The prevalence of congenital inverted nipple. *Aesthetic Plastic Surgery, 23,* 144-146.

Pawson, E.G., & Petrakis, N.L. (1975). Comparison of breast pigmentation among women of different racial groups. *Human Biology, 47,* 441-450.

Perez-Izquierdo, J., Vilata, J., Sanchez, J., Gargallo, E., Millan, F., & Aliaga, A. (1990). Retinoic treatment of nipple hyperkeratosis. *Archives of Dermatology, 126,* 687-688.

Perkins, O.C., & Miller, A.M. (1926). Sebaceous glands in the human nipple. *American Journal of Obstetrics and Gynecology, 11,* 789-794.

Peters, F., Diemer, P., Mecks, O., & Behnken, L.J. (2003). Severity of mastalgia in relation to milk duct dilatation. *Obstetrics and Gynecology, 101*, 54–60.

Pfaller, M.A. (1994). Epidemiology and control of fungal infections. *Clinical Infectious Disease, 19* (S1), S8–S13.

Piatt, J.P., & Bergeson, P.S. (1992). Gentian violet toxicity. *Clinical Pediatrics, 31*, 756–757.

Pizzo, G., Giuliana, G., Milici, M.E., & Giangreco, R. (2000). Effects of dietary carbohydrate on the in vitro epithelial adhesion of *Candida albicans, Candida tropicalis*, and *Candida krusei. New Microbiology, 23*, 63–71.

Porter, J., & Schach, B. (2004). Treating sore, possibly infected nipples. *Journal of Human Lactation, 20,* 221-222.

Porter, R.H., & Winberg, J. (1999). Unique salience of maternal breast odors for newborn infants. *Neuroscience Biobehavior Review, 23*, 439-449.

Proctor, R.A., von Eiff, C., Kahl, B.C., Becker, K., McNamara, P., Herrmann, M., & Peters, G. (2006). Small colony variants: A pathogenic form of bacteria that facilitates persistent and recurrent infections. *Nature Reviews Microbiology, 4,* 295-305.

Pugh, L.C., Buchko, B.L., Bishop, B.A., Cochran, J.F., Smith, L.R., & Lerew, D.J. (1996). A comparison of topical agents to relieve nipple pain and enhance breastfeeding. *Birth, 23*, 88-93.

Rago, J.L. (1988). Weeping areolar eczema. *Journal of Human Lactation, 4*,166–167.

Rahal, R.M., deFreitas-Junior, R., & Paulinelli, R.R. (2005). Risk factors for duct ectasia. *Breast Journal, 11*, 262-265.

Rahbar, F. (1982). Clinical significance of supernumerary nipples in black neonates. *Clinical Pediatrics, 21*, 46-47.

Ramirez, O.M. (2002). Reduction mammaplasty with the "owl" incision and no undermining. *Plastic Reconstructive Surgery, 109*, 512–522.

Ramsay, D.T., Kent, J.C., Hartmann, R.A., & Hartmann, P.E. (2005). Anatomy of the lactating breast redefined with ultrasound imaging. *Journal of Anatomy, 206*, 525–534.

Reilly, A., & Snyder, B. (2005). Raynaud's phenomenon: Whether it's primary or secondary, there is no cure, but treatment can alleviate symptoms. *American Journal of Nursing, 105*, 56-65.

Remington, J.S., & Klein, J.O. (1983). *Infectious diseases of the fetus and newborn.* Philadelphia, PA: WB Saunders.

Renfrew, M.J., Woolridge, M.W., & McGill, H.R. (2000). *Enabling women to breastfeed: A review of practices which promote or inhibit breastfeeding—with evidence-based guidance for practice.* London: The Stationary Office.

Righard, L. (1996). Early enhancement of successful breastfeeding. *World Health Forum, 17,* 92–97.

Righard, L. (1998). Are breastfeeding problems related to incorrect breastfeeding technique and the use of pacifiers and bottles? *Birth, 25*, 40–44.

Riordan, J. (1985). The effectiveness of topical agents in reducing nipple soreness of breastfeeding mothers. *Journal of Human Lactation, 1*, 36-41.

Robins, A. (1991). *Biological perspectives on human pigmentation.* New York: Cambridge University Press.

Robinson, L.B. (2002). Olive oil: A natural treatment for sore nipples? *AWHONN Lifelines, 6*, 110-112.

Rosa, C., Novak, F.R., Almeida, J.A.G., Hagler, L.C., & Hagler, A.N. (1990). Yeasts from human milk collected in Rio de Janeiro, Brazil. Review. *Microbiology, 21*, 361–363.

Rusby, J.E., Brachterl, E.F., Michaelson, J.S., Koerner, F.C., & Smith, B.L . (2007). Breast duct anatomy in the human nipple: Three-dimensional patterns and clinical implications. *Breast Cancer Research Treatment, 106*, 171-179.

Russell, M.J. (1976). Human olfactory communication. *Nature, 260*, 520-522.

Ryan, T.J. (2007). Infection following soft tissue injury: Its role in wound healing. *Current Opinion in Infectious Disease, 20*, 124-128.

Saary, J., Querishi, R., Palda, V., DeKoven, J., Pratt, M., Skotnicki-Grant, S., et al. (2005). A systematic review of contact dermatitis treatment and prevention. *Journal of the American Academy of Dermatology, 53*, 845.e1-845.e13.

Sadove, R., & Clayman, M.A. (2008). Surgical procedure for reversal of nipple piercing. *Aesthetic Plastic Surgery, 32*, 563-565.

Sakazaki, F., Kataoka, H., Okuno, T., Ueno, H., Semma, M., Ichikawa, A., et al. (2007). Ozonated olive oil enhances the growth of granulation tissue in a mouse model of pressure ulcer. *Ozone: Science & Engineering, 29*, 503-507.

Sanuki. J., Fukama, E., & Uchida, Y. (2008). Morphologic study of nipple-areola complex in 600 breasts. *Aesthetic Plastic Surgery, 33*, 295-297.

Sarhadi, N.S., Shaw Dunn, J., Lee, F.D., & Soutar, D.S. (1996). An anatomical study of the nerve supply of the breast, including the nipple and areola. *British Journal of Plastic Surgery, 49*, 156-164.

Schaal, B. (1986). Presumed olfactory exchanges between mother and neonate in humans. In J. Le Camus & J. Cosnier (Eds.), *Ethology and psychology* (pp.101-110). Toulouse: Privat, I.E.C.

Schaal, B., Coureaud, G., Doucet, S., Delaunay-El Allam, M., Moncomble, A.S., Montigny, D., et al. (2009). Mammary olfactory signalization in females and odor processing in neonates: Ways evolved by rabbits and humans. *Behavior*

Brain Research, 200, 346-358.

Schaal, B., Doucet, S., Sagot, P., Hertling, E., & Soussignan, R. (2006). Human breast areolae as scent organs: Morphological data and possible involvement in maternal-neonatal coadaptation. *Developmental Psychobiology, 48*, 100-110.

Schelz, Z., Molnar, J., & Hohmann, J. (2006). Antimicrobial and antiplasmid activities of essential oils. *Fitoterapia, 77*, 279-285.

Schlenz, I., Kuzbari, R., Gruber, H., & Holle, J. (2000). The sensitivity of the nipple-areola complex: An anatomic study. *Plastic Reconstructive Surgery, 105*, 905–909.

Schwartz, K., D'Arcy, H.J., Gillespie, B., Bobo, J., Longeway, M., & Foxman, B . (2002). Factors associated with weaning in the first 3 months postpartum. *Journal of Family Practice, 51*, 439–444.

Sealander, J.Y., & Kerr, C.P. (1989). Herpes simplex of the nipple: infant-to-mother transmission. *American Family Physician, 39*, 111-113.

Servili, M., Esposto, S., Fabiani, R., Urbani, S., Taticchi, A., Mariucci, F., et al. (2009). Phenolic compounds in olive oil: Antioxidant, health and organoleptic activities according to their chemical structure. *Inflammopharmacology, 17*, 76-84.

Sharp, D.A. (1992). Moist wound healing for sore or cracked nipples. *Breastfeeding Abstracts, 12*, 19.

Shastry, V., Betkerur, J., & Kushalappa, P.A. (2006). Unilateral nevoid hyperkeratosis of the nipple: A report of two cases. *Indian Journal of Dermatology, Venereology, Leprology, 72*, 303-305.

Smith, W.L., Erenberg, A., & Nowak, A. (1988). Imaging evaluation of the human nipple during breastfeeding. *American Journal of Diseases in Children, 142*, 76-78.

Smith, W.L., Erenberg, A., Nowak, A., & Franken, E.A. (1985). Physiology of sucking in the normal term infant using real-time. *U.S. Radiology, 156*, 379-381.

Soukka, T., Tenovuo, J., & Lenander-Lemikari, M. (1992). Fungicidal effect of human lactoferrin against *Candida albicans. FEMS Microbiology Letter, 69*, 223–228.

Spangler, A., & Hildebrandt, E. (1993). The effect of modified lanolin on nipple pain/damage during the first ten days of breastfeeding. *International Journal of Childbirth Education, 8*, 15-19.

Srinivasan, A., Dobrich, C., Mitnick, H., & Feldman, P. (2006). Ankyloglossia in breastfeeding infants: The effect of frenotomy on maternal nipple pain and latch. *Breastfeeding Medicine, 1*, 216-224.

Staib, P., Kretschmar, M., Nichterlein, T., Hof, H., & Morschhäuser, J. (2000). Differential activation of a *Candida albicans* virulence gene family during infection. *Proceedings of the National Academy of Science, 97,* 6102–6107.

Stewart, P.S., & Costerton, J.W. (2001). Antibiotic resistance of bacteria in biofilms. *Lancet, 358(9276),* 135-138.

Storr, G.B. (1988). Prevention of nipple tenderness and breast engorgement in the postpartal period. *Journal of Obstetric, Gynecologic and Neonatal Nursing, 17,* 203-209.

Strom, S.S., Baldwin, B.J., Sigurdson, A.J., & Schusterman, M.A. (1997). Cosmetic saline breast implants: A survey of satisfaction, breastfeeding experience, cancer screening, and health. *Plastic Reconstructive Surgery, 100,* 1553–1557.

Sullivan-Bolyai, J.Z., Fife, K.H., Jacobs, R.F., Miller, Z., & Corey, L. (1983). Disseminated neonatal herpes simplex virus type 1 from a maternal breast lesion. *Pediatrics, 71,* 455–457.

Taneri, F., Kurukahvecioglu, O., Akyurek, N., Tekin, E.H., Ilhan, M.N., Cifter, C., et al. (2006). Microanatomy of milk ducts in the nipple. *European Surgical Research, 38,* 545–549.

Tanquay, K., McBean, M., & Jain, E. (1994). Nipple candidosis among breastfeeding mothers: A case control study of predisposing factors. *Canadian Family Physician, 40,* 1407–1413.

Tedeschi, L., Ahari, S., Byrne, J. (1963). Involutional mammary duct ectasia and periductal mastitis. *American Journal of Surgery, 106,* 517–521.

Terrill, P.J., & Stapleton, M.J. (1991). The inverted nipple: To cut the ducts or not? *British Journal of Plastic Surgery, 44,* 372–377.

Thomassen, P., Johansson, V.A, Wassberg, C., & Petrini, B. (1998). Breastfeeding, pain and infection. *Gynecology Obstetric Investigation, 46,* 73–74.

Thorley, V. (1997). Inverted nipple with fatty plaques on areola and nipple. *Breastfeeding Review, 5,* 43–44.

Turner, T.D. (1979). Hospital usage of absorbent dressings. *Pharmacology Journal, 222,* 421-426.

Utter, A.R. (1990). Gentian violet treatment for thrush: Can its use cause breastfeeding problems? (letter). *Journal of Human Lactation, 6,* 178–180.

Utter, A.R. (1992). Gentian violet and thrush (letter). *Journal of Human Lactation, 8,* 6.

Uvnas-Moberg, K., & Eriksson, M. (1996). Breastfeeding: Physiological, endocrine and behavioral adaptations caused by oxytocin and local neurogenic activity in the nipple and mammary gland. *Acta Paediatrica, 85,* 525-530.

Varendi, H., Porter, R.H., & Winberg, J. (1994). Does the newborn baby find the nipple by smell? *Lancet, 344,* 989-990.

Varsano, I.B., Jaber, L., Garty, B.Z., Mukamel, M.M., & Grünebaum, M. (1984). Urinary tract abnormalities in children with supernumerary nipples. *Pediatrics,*

73, 103-105.

Vazirinejad, R., Darakhshan, S., Esmaeili, A., & Hadadian, S. (2009). The effect of maternal breast variations on neonatal weight gain in the first seven days of life. *International Breastfeeding Journal, 4*, 13.

Vidotto, B., Guevara-Ochoa, L., Ponce, L.M., Tello, G.M., Prada, G.R., & Bruatto, M. (1992). Vaginal yeast flora of pregnant women in the Cusco region of Peru. *Mycoses, 35*, 229–234.

Von Eiff, C., Peters, G., & Becker, K. The small colony variant (SCV) concept - The role of staphylococcal SCVs in persistent infections. *Injury, 37*, S26-S33.

Vuorenkoski, V., Wasz-Hockert, O., Koivisto, E., & Lind, J. (1969). The effect of cry stimulus on the temperature of the lactating breast of primipara. *Experientia, 25*, 1286-1287.

Walker, M., & Driscoll, J.W. (1989). Sore nipples: The new mother's nemesis. *American Journal of Maternal Child Nursing, 14*, 260–265.

Wallace, H., & Clark, S. (2006). Tongue tie division in infants with breastfeeding difficulties. *International Journal of Pediatric Otorhinolaryngology, 70*, 1257-1261.

Waller, H.K. (1938). *Clinical studies in lactation.* Heinemann Ltd.

Waller, H.K. (1943). A reflex governing the outflow of milk from the breast. *Lancet, 241(6229)*, 69-71.

Waller, H.K. (1946). The early failure of breastfeeding: A clinical study of its causes and their prevention. *Archives of Disease in Children, 21*, 1-12.

Waller, H.K. (1947). Some clinical aspects of lactation. *Archives of Disease in Children, 22*, 193-199.

Wambach, K.A., & Koehn, M. (2004). Experiences of infant-feeding decision-making among urban economically disadvantaged pregnant adolescents. *Journal of Advanced Nursing, 48*, 361-370.

Ward, K.A., & Burton, J.L. (1997). Dermatologic diseases of the breast in young women. *Clinical Dermatology, 15*, 45–52.

Weber, F., Woolridge, M.W., & Baum, J.D. (1986). An ultrasonographic study of the organization of sucking and swallowing by newborn infants. *Developmental Medicine and Child Neurology, 28*, 19-24.

West, D., & Hirsch, E.M. (2008).*Breastfeeding after breast and nipple procedures: A guide for healthcare professionals*. Amarillo, TX: Hale Publishing.

West, C. (1980). Factors influencing the duration of breastfeeding. *Journal of Biosocial Science, 12*, 325–331.

Whitley, N. (1978). Preparation for breastfeeding: A one year follow-up of 34 nursing mothers. *Journal of Obstetric Gynecologic and Neonatal Nursing, 7*,

44-48.

Widstrom, A.M, & Thingstrom-Paulsson, J. (1993). The position of the tongue during rooting reflexes elicited in newborn infants before the first suckle. *Acta Paediatrica Scandinavia, 82,* 281–283.

Wiechula, R. (2003). The use of moist wound-healing dressings in the management of split-thickness skin graft donor sites: A systematic review. *International Journal of Nursing Practice, 9,* S9-S17.

Wiener, S. (2006). Diagnosis and management of Candida of the nipple and breast. *Journal of Midwifery and Women's Health, 51,* 125-128.

Wilson-Clay, B. (2003). Nipple shields in clinical practice: A review. *Breastfeeding Abstracts, 22,* 11–12.

Wilson-Clay, B., & Hoover, K. (2008). *The breastfeeding atlas.* 4th ed. Austin, TX: LactNews Press.

Winter, G.D. (1962). Formation of scab and rate of epithelialization of superficial wounds in the skin of the young domestic pig. *Nature, 193,* 293-294.

Woolridge, M.W. (1986a). The 'anatomy' of infant sucking. *Midwifery, 2,* 164-171.

Woolridge, M.W. (1986b). Aetiology of sore nipples. *Midwifery, 2,* 172–176.

Yeung, D., Pennell, M., Leung, M., & Hall, J. (1981). Breastfeeding: Prevalence and influencing factors. *Canadian Journal of Public Health, 72,* 323–330.

Ziemer, M.M., Cooper, D.M., & Pigeon, J.G. (1995). Evaluation of a dressing to reduce nipple pain and improve nipple skin condition in breastfeeding women. *Nursing Research, 44,* 347–351.

Ziemer, M.M., Paone, J.P., Schupay, J., & Cole, E. (1990). Methods to prevent and manage nipple pain in breastfeeding women. *Western Journal of Nursing Research, 12,* 732-744.

Ziemer, M.M., & Pigeon, J.G. (1993). Skin changes and pain in the nipple during the 1st week of lactation. *Journal of Obstetric Gynecologic Neonatal Nursing, 22,* 247–256.

Zollner, M., & Jorge, A. (2003). Candida spp. Occurrence in oral cavities of breastfeeding infants and in their mothers' mouths and breasts. *Pesquisa Odontológica Brasileira, 17,* 151-155.

INDEX

AUTHOR BIOGRAPHY

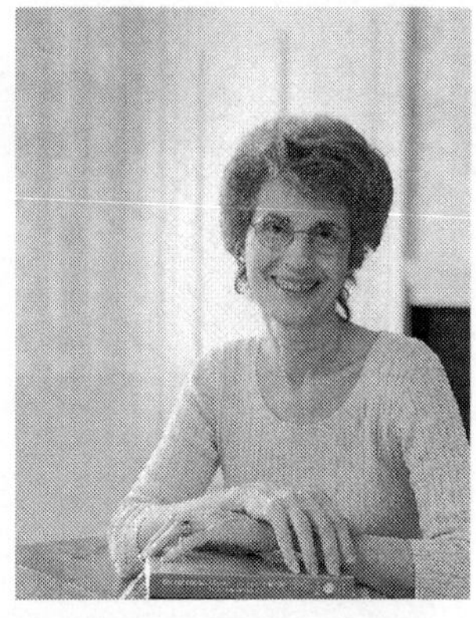

Marsha Walker, RN, IBCLC is the Executive Director of the National Alliance for Breastfeeding Advocacy, Research, Education and Legal Branch (NABA REAL). She is a long time breastfeeding advocate, starting as a volunteer breastfeeding counselor with the Nursing Mothers Counsel in California. Marsha went on to become a childbirth educator through Lamaze International, a registered nurse, and an International Board Certified Lactation Consultant. She served on the Representative Panel of Experts in 1985, which constructed the first lactation consultant exam and was one of a number of clinicians on whose practice the exam grid is based. Marsha enjoyed a large clinical lactation practice at Harvard Pilgrim Health Plan, a major HMO in Massachusetts, where she was the Director of the Breastfeeding Support Program for 12 years. She has served on the Board of Directors of the International Lactation Consultant Association (ILCA) for seven years, including as its president in 1999.

Marsha is on the Board of Directors of the Massachusetts Breastfeeding Coalition, Baby Friendly USA, the U.S. Lactation Consultant Association, and Best for Babes. She is ILCA's representative to the U.S. Department of Agriculture's Breastfeeding Promotion Consortium and NABA's representative to the U.S. Breastfeeding Committee. She has worked for eight years to get breastfeeding legislation passed in her state of Massachusetts, which became a reality in January 2009. She is the co-chair of the Ban the Bags campaign, a national effort to eliminate the hospital distribution of formula company discharge bags.

NABA REAL is the IBFAN organization in the United States and is responsible for monitoring the International Code of Marketing of Breastmilk Substitutes in the U.S. Marsha has written both country reports on Code monitoring activities in the U.S., *Selling Out Mothers and Babies* and *Still Selling Out Mothers and Babies*. Marsha is an international speaker on breastfeeding and an author of numerous publications, including her book, *Breastfeeding Management for the Clinician: Using the Evidence.*

Marsha is married and the mother of two breastfed children, Shannon (33) and Justin (32), her original breastfeeding clinical instructors. She is the grandmother of 4 breastfed girls: Haley, Sophie, Isabelle, and Ella.

Printed in Great Britain
by Amazon